THE PSYCHOLOGY
OF CANCER

WHY WE GET CANCER. HOW TO FIGHT IT.
WHAT IT CAN TEACH US

KEITH SCOTT-MUMBY MD, MB ChB, HMD, PhD

Published by Mother Whale Inc.
8550 W Charleston Bldv.
Suite 102-160
Las Vegas, NV 89117

ISBN STUFF

First edition.
1 2 3 4 5 6 7 8 9 10

Design and layout by Dragos Balasoiu
(contact@dragosb.com)

DISCLAIMER

Publisher's and author's note:

This book is intended as a reference volume only, not as a medical manual. The ideas, procedures and suggestions contained herein are not intended as a substitute for consulting with your personal medical practitioner. Neither the publisher nor the author shall be liable for any loss or damage allegedly arising from any information or suggestions in this book, howsoever applied or misapplied. Further, if you have a medical problem, we urge you to seek advice from a licensed medical practitioner.

Through the millennia, humanity has more or less consciously known that all diseases ultimately have a psychic origin and it became a "scientific" asset firmly anchored in the inheritance of universal knowledge; it is only modern medicine that has turned our animated beings into a bag full of chemical formulas.

- Reike Geerd Hamer MD

Life is 10% what happens to me and 90% how I react to it.

- Charles Swindoll, pastor and preacher.

CONTENTS

WHAT CANCER CAN TEACH US

DOES PRAYER HELP? YOU BET!

CANCER PSYCHOLOGY

WHY WE GET CANCER. HOW TO FIGHT IT. WHAT IT CAN TEACH US.

AM I GOING TO DIE?

Cancer will bring you up against the issue of your mortality for sure. Even the most slow-growing cancer will still scare the victim who hears those words, "It's bad news I'm afraid..." For that reason alone, life often takes on a completely new direction after the diagnosis. It's not all bad and we are going to explore that. Some people have even told us that they were *glad* they got cancer, because it brought so many important and positive changes to a life which was, up to that point, aimlessly drifting along.

Mass entertainments, sugary food and drinks, slouching around watching TV and chemical highs are not really helpful towards the ideal and healthy human life. Maybe you don't live like that; most do! It needs to change. So the first keynote psychological improvement is made in a split second: the decision to get out of the lazy, comfortable rut of modern living. Not that it means adopting a life of sackcloth, ashes and self-punishment. It just means getting off the bus to nowhere and finding your real destination in life!

When the diagnosis of cancer is made, the patient typically goes through five classic stages of trauma and loss described by Elisabeth Kübler-Ross (which is the correct spelling).

Kübler-Ross pioneered methods in the support and counseling of personal trauma, grief and grieving, associated with death and dying. She also dramatically improved the understanding and practices in relation to bereavement and hospice care. This is quite aside from the validity of her theoretical work itself.

Whether grieving for ourselves (the patient) or for a loved one who is faced with a potentially-terminal illness, there is what Dr. Kübler-Ross called a "grief cycle".

It has five stages, notably denial, anger, bargaining, depression, and finally acceptance. Here it is in brief:

Stage 1. Denial	Refusal to accept the facts. It can't be true...
Stage 2. Anger	There is protest, rejection and rage...
Stage 3. Bargaining	Trying to work some way out of the dilemma or pain, deals with God, if I do this... etc.
Stage 4. Depression	The person is gradually moving over to grieving. He or she has begun to face the inevitability.
Stage 5. Acceptance	Depending on the person and the situation, he or she becomes detached and objective.

The Grief Cycle first published in *On Death and Dying*, Elisabeth Kübler-Ross, 1969

Well, I'm here to tell you this: famous as it is, and although valid in its way, the Grief Cycle is not your only choice and certainly not your best choice. Let's call it the "Inevitability" pathway.

But how about the: "Fight It Every Inch Of The Way" pathway? The thing is, cancer can be beaten. With or without orthodox treatment, millions of people have beaten the rap. **Cancer is not a death knell**, has been one of my key mottoes these forty years. It's a wake up call, telling you that your health is in ruins. But it is unlikely to kill you if you take the right effective action.

So wake up!

As will be revealed to you when you read on, the patients who do best are those who refuse to accept they are going down, won't listen to predictions that they are going to die, now or any time soon, and often yap and snarl at the doctor for his defeatist incompetence.

Successful (survivor) patients take control of the threatening situation; they become their own case manager; they hire and fire a team of supporters; and woe-betide anyone in their proximity who thinks negatively!

Under no circumstances leave your treatment program to your oncologist. The silly belief that he or she is the "expert" and knows everything about cancer will get you laid in your grave before you know it.

By all means listen to their information, adapt what is useful, choose your treatment wisely and do not be bullied or railroaded into their wishes. They are just there to make money. It sounds cynical, but everyone works at a job, to pay for a home, buy food, take vacations and generally support their family. You know it's true. The mere fact that an oncologist has chosen to treat cancers as a lucrative way of making money should not impress you and certainly not lead you to believe he or she is some kind of angel with miraculous insight into health and disease.

In fact they are a pretty ignorant bunch, who ignore lifestyle factors such as diet and nutrition, underplay the uselessness of what they do and consider anyone who teaches body wisdom as some kind of crank or, if medically trained, a quack.

You have been warned.

Back To School

There is nothing an oncologist hates more than an informed patient who keeps asking difficult questions, won't do just as they are told and subsequently refuses to die on schedule. It drives them crazy (good!)

But really, knowledge is going to save your life. Ignorance will likely end it.

If you cannot get information from your oncologist, where will you find it? The Internet is very tempting. But let me caution you that the Internet is not policed and there are rogues out there, peddling crackpot—even dangerous—opinions, substances and techniques, who want your money. Just because he or she claims to be in the holistic field, don't be fooled into thinking he or she is sweetness and light and would not tell a lie.

Greed is everywhere and in many different guises.

Also beware that many holistic practitioners, or health researchers as they like to call themselves, are medically not qualified at all and don't even have a first aid certificate. Yet they presume to tell you how to conquer one of the most dangerous of all maladies. Many have fine looking websites and lots of testimonials. What you don't get is how many of their cases died or abandoned the program, compared to those with a nice inspiring testimonial.

At the risk of further alarming or depressing you, let me tell you that there are websites out there where—for a fee—someone will record a hearty testimonial saying pretty much anything the customer asks for.

So be careful.

At the end, I'll give you some trusted websites, where the great bulk of the information given is reliable and effective. Till then, let's work on the basics. Deal?

LIFE IS OFTEN THE DISEASE, CANCER THE RESULT

Disease won't touch you if you are happy and zestfully healthy.

In a sense, you could say that the actual disease is the patient's life! The illness the patient is experiencing is simply the result of all the many problems and indiscretions that are wrong with his or her life.

By that, I don't just mean the obvious things, such as diet, smoking and stress. These are important issues, naturally. But there are in addition the numerous factors in our day-to-day living experience which can go wrong and cause us to suffer. Such adversities can be as broad as financial hardship, poor relationships, pressure at school or work, lack of sleep, bereavement, emotional instability or just plain "overdoing things".

It is wrong for doctors to concentrate merely on the manifestation of the disease process. It is a very late development. One only becomes ill after the compensation mechanisms have broken down. After all, our bodies protect us from certain death every day--- we wouldn't last more than a few hours or days at most without them. It is the failure of this defensive process that is the real cause of illness. To label a condition "cancer" is to entirely mislead self and others as to the true nature of what is going on. It should be "a progressive dysfunction of body mechanisms *resulting* in cancer".

Notice the word progressive, which is crucial. You can't get to a disease state in one jump from being healthy! Even the terrible killer Black Death only killed a proportion of the population--- basically those who were ready for it. Disease won't touch you if you are happy and zestfully healthy. If only medical students were taught this simple truth in letters of fire, we would have a sympathetic and enlightened medical profession that did not attract to itself the same opprobrium and scorn that it tends to today.

I go along with Sondra Ray's wise words:

"What do you do when your body starts acting up or breaking down, or gets a sore, a pain, a fracture, an infection? As you know the wisest course of action is to take care of it right away. What happens if you don't? Chances are your body won't heal. What if you still don't pay attention? It may very likely get worse and worse, until you have a full-blown disease. If on the other hand you are careful to heal each problem as it comes up, you can stay healthy. Your body can work. And if you live a healthy lifestyle, eating well, preventing pains, illnesses, and tensions, that is even better. You are enjoying the vitality of life. You master our own body and feel great.

"What I'm saying is this: when we're dealing with our relationships and our bodies, we must look at the writing on the wall. We must identify what is off balance right now and handle it before it is too late.

> "This may sound like nothing more than simple, common sense. But it's often wise to rely on your common sense and act on it. How committed are you to living fully, one hundred percent of the time? Are you actually more committed to mediocrity, suffering, suppression, pain, lack of joy and failure? My hunch is that you would prefer joy, excellence, and pleasure. Once you get a taste of how it feels to live a cleaned-up life, you won't want to tolerate the old ways of living much longer." (*Loving Relationships: II*, Celestial Arts, 1995, p. 84)

Be warned because we can "clean up your life" with Supernoetics® mentoring and piloting (healing of memory and life hurts). Let's go for joy, excellence and pleasure!

Cancer will bounce off us like a rubber ball hitting a solid wall!

CONTEXT

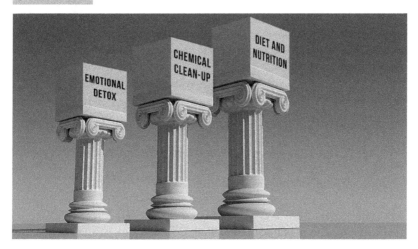

Without question, diet and nutrition is the number one pillar. It is unarguable that among native, "primitive" or paleolithic societies, who retain their natural diet, cancer is completely unknown.

Harvard anthropologist and Arctic explorer Vilhjalmur Stefansson spent more than 30 seasons among the Canadian Inuit eskimos and reports that he never saw a single case of cancer. He wrote a book covering his research, entitled *Cancer: disease of civilization?: An anthropological and historical study* (1960).

Nobel Peace Prize Laureate Albert Schweitzer reported much the same thing. He spent decades living in the Gabon, among African natives. There was no cancer among those who adhered to their natural diet.

Chemical clean-up is pillar number 2. To date there have been a conservative one million chemical compounds developed which are not natural and therefore potentially carcinogenic (cancer causing). There are currently some 80,000 of those substances still in manufacture, the vast majority of which have never been properly evaluated for safety. Your body is awash with potentially carcinogenic substances: cleaners, cosmetics, solvents, paints, cosmetics, drugs, synthetic hormones, food additives and more.

We are living in what I call a "chemical blizzard". You need to take steps to clean up your personal local environment. That's another book entirely. Try Dr. Doris Rapp's best-selling book *Our Toxic World, A Wake Up Call* (Environmental Medical Research Foundation, Buffalo, NY, 2003).

The third and usually-forgotten pillar is arguably the most important and that is the **Pillar of Emotional Detoxing**. As an internationally-known holistic health expert, I find people engaging in all sorts of therapies and practices to try to beat cancer. They will juice, meditate, pray, take supplements, seek out oxygen therapy, colonic irrigation, hitch themselves up to electronic machines, undergo vigorous diet regimes, such as the Gerson Therapy, the Kelley Program and the Budwig diet... You name it, nothing is too extreme to try.

But these same people will avoid any emotional issue to the death. I mean literally to the death: I saw one woman beat cancer twice, using the Gerson Protocol, which is pretty drastic—so much so that I warn people it is virtually a career shift—yet she would not listen when I told her she must get her hidden emotional issues fixed. She did not listen, played it down, and the third time she came to see me it was too late—her lungs were riddled with metastases and already filling up with fluid.

"I don't have any hidden emotional issues," is one common attitude. Perhaps even more common is "It was an issue but I've dealt with it." Dealt with it? When you are on a pathway to death?

I don't think so.

Anyway, you now understand the immense importance I give to emotional detoxing and—on the positive side—to the positive role of the mind in healing.

So, let's get down to work...

This Book

This text is divided into three principal sections:

1. Psychological reasons we may attract cancer

2. Vigorous psychological changes that must be undertaken, to significantly improve your chances of beating it; and finally,

3. How to use what you have learned on your journey to create a new, healthy and beautiful second life for yourself.

What will not be covered:

a. Diet and nutrition
b. Chemical burdens
c. So-called "chemo brain"
d. Genetic factors (except to separate them from hereditary influences)
e. Special or general health remedies, herbs, substances or medicines
f. Otto Warburg's oxygen theory
g. Viral causes of cancer
h. Rife machines and electronic devices (zappers, etc.)
i. Crank ideas, like the Marshall protocol
j. Brilliant new innovations in orthodox medicine (where we work with the immune system, instead of destroying it).

I built my reputation on being a person of integrity, who reports facts with the support of scientific research and published studies. I have endeavored, throughout this present work, to enrich the text with a number of citations. Nevertheless, it can be hard at times to decide what the literature is really struggling to say; it's rarely unequivocal.

Beyond everyday science, a special section has been reserved for the consideration of spiritual healing, transcendental phenomena and "miracles", called *Where Is God In All This?* (page 105 onwards)

Essentially, *The Psychology Of Cancer* concentrates solely on the mind as a causative and healing factor in the development of and recovery from cancer.

It is a how-to manual. Just reading this book will not save you. Getting to grips with the issues it raises and properly solving them may very well do so however.

PART 1

WHY DO WE GET CANCERS?

Does the way you think, feel and behave have any connection with why you get sick? It certainly does.

I've been teaching it for over 40 years, but we are only beginning to understand, *in a scientific way*, the connection between disease and the mind. There is a rapidly growing body of research studying the relationship between emotions, personality characteristics, and disease, especially cancer. The answers are beginning to emerge, and they demonstrate a definite connection between emotions and the chances of developing cancer, as well as the prognosis of the disease once it has appeared. This short text will help you to understand the most recent developments and discoveries.

Historically, this idea of emotions influencing cancer goes back a very l-o-n-g way. Galen (130-200 AD), a prominent Greek physician, surgeon and philosopher in the Roman Empire, famously remarked, "Cancer does not strike a happy person."

Actually, he didn't quite say that! He said, cancer is caused by an excess of black bile. Black bile is another way of saying *melancholic,* which means depressed and despondent.

[Incidentally, Galen gave us the word *oncos* (Greek for swelling) to describe tumors; hence *oncology*].

We no longer use the black bile, yellow bile, blood and phlegm model. Instead we have the science of psychology. Several personality characteristics appear to influence the course of cancer: depression, stress, lacking a sense of control, having a negative outlook, and lacking an adequate support system.

If there is something broken in your emotional make up, that will probably flag up a poor prognosis. Having a sense of control, a positive outlook, and a good support system all correlate with a better prognosis.

This is not just a claim. There is science behind the idea. While negative emotions predict a poorer prognosis for cancer patients, positive feelings like joy go together with a better outcome. For example, a seven-year follow-up of breast cancer patients by Sandra Levy, associate professor of psychiatry and medicine at the University of Pittsburgh and director of behavioral medicine in oncology at the Pittsburgh Cancer Institute, showed that those patients who expressed more joy in their lives when initially tested lived longer. This result does not conflict with other studies that showed that an angry or fighting response to cancer predicts a better outcome. It is quite possible to have a sense of joy in life and a fighting spirit at the same time.

Optimism helps too. A study of women with cervical cell abnormalities reported that the women with high scores for pessimism, hopelessness, and social alienation were more likely to progress to cancer of the cervix. On the other hand, optimism and active coping styles were connected with reduced risk of progress to cancer.

Of course we must not forget that the diagnosis of cancer itself is extremely traumatic and depressing. According to a study led by Ludwig-Maximilians-Universitaet (LMU) in Munich, a majority of patients diagnosed with breast cancer go on to develop symptoms of post-traumatic stress disorder, and in most of these cases the symptoms persist for at least a year.

During the interval between diagnosis of cancer and the initiation of treatment, 82.5% of all patients were found to exhibit symptoms of Post Traumatic Stress Disorder (PTSD), such as recurrent and intrusive reminders of the experiences associated with cancer, feelings of detachment and emotional numbness, increased arousal, sudden outbursts of anger and an exaggerated startle response.

Although a full diagnosis of PTSD was found in only 2% of patients one year after the cancer diagnosis, more than half (57.3%) continued to display one or more significant symptoms of PTSD at that point.

Does PTSD Cause Cancer?

An obvious question follows: if stress is a significant contributor to developing cancer, then PTSD must surely be a major risk factor?

In fact that seems not to be the case. Cancer can result in PTSD, at least temporarily, but does not arise any more frequently in the general population than is PTSD victims.

In the largest study to date that examines Post Traumatic Stress Disorder as a risk factor for cancer, researchers from Boston University School of Medicine (BUSM), have shown no evidence of an association.

Researchers compared the rate of various cancer diagnoses among people with PTSD with the standardized cancer rate from the general population in the same time period using data from the Danish national medical and social registers. They found PTSD was not associated with an increased risk for cancer.

"The general public may have a perception that stress contributes to cancer occurrence and given the ubiquity of PTSD and cancer and their costs to individuals and society, any observed associations could have meaningful public health implications," explained co-author Jaimie L. Gradus, DSc, MPH, assistant professor of psychiatry and epidemiology at BUSM and an epidemiologist at the National Center for PTSD. "This study, however, provided no evidence that a severe chronic stress disorder such as PTSD is associated with cancer incidence."

[Jaimie L. Gradus, Dóra Körmendiné Farkas, Elisabeth Svensson, Vera Ehrenstein, Timothy L. Lash, Arnold Milstein, Nancy Adler, Henrik Toft Sørensen. Posttraumatic stress disorder and cancer risk: a nationwide cohort study. European Journal of Epidemiology, 2015; DOI: 10.1007/s10654-015-0032-7]

Stress And Cancer

The previously-quoted study does not mean that stress, per se, is not a contributor to cancer. It most certainly is. Perhaps PTSD is a special kind of psychological syndrome, with its own "rules".

Later on we shall see that measures of stress can predict the onset of many diseases, of which cancer is just one (page 22 Hamer and Holmes-Rahe)

Several studies have shown that chronic stress exerts a general immuno-suppressive effect that suppresses or withholds the body's ability to initiate a prompt, efficient immune reaction [Hafen BQ, Frandsen KJ, Karren K, Hooker KR. The health effects of attitudes, emotions and relationships. Provo UT: EMS Associates; 1991 and [Huebner HS. Burnout among school psychologists: An exploratory investigation into its nature, extent and correlates. School Psychol Quart. 1992;7:129–36]

Most sensible physicians view cancer as primarily a disease of the immune system: the so-called "surveillance model" (see below).

The relationship between breast cancer and stress has received particular attention in recent years. Some studies of breast cancer rates have shown significantly high incidence of disease among those women who experienced traumatic life events and losses within a few years of their diagnosis.

The argument sometimes arises that most cancers have been developing for years and are diagnosed only after they have been growing in the body for a long time. Therefore the time association between the death of a loved one and the triggering of cancer doesn't hold. I say this is pure speculation. If the cancer was unknown prior to diagnosis, who can say what it was doing or how fast it was growing? Not logical, as Mr. Spock would say.

There are continuing claims that there is no scientific evidence that stress-induced changes in the immune system directly cause cancer (not true, as you will see). But in any case, that's to miss another important question: whether there is a relationship between psychological stress and the transformation of normal cells into cancerous cells?

It's odd the way doctors and researchers just ignore studies that seem to contradict their pet theories. There is a whole army of people (oncologists and radiologists in particular) who obsessively seem to want to debunk the role of the mind in disease and the power of the mind in healing.

We can steer the other way and welcome evidence showing that how you feel, what you think and how you behave has an influence on your entire make up!

Studies in animals, mostly rats, revealed the link between stress and progression of cancerous tumors. Chronic and acute stress, including surgery and social disruptions, appear to promote tumor growth. It is easy to do such research in animals, but it is harder with humans, that's true. Researchers cannot expose people to tumor cells to see what happens, as they do with animals. Furthermore, there are many systems that affect cancer, from the immune system to the endocrine system, along with environment factors that are impossible to control for, which makes sorting out the role of the stress element extremely difficult.

A 1999 study [Azar B. Probing links between stress and cancer. APA Monitor Online. 1999;30:1–4. (http://www.apa.org/monitor/jun99/stress.html] found that there was a link between stress, tumor development and a type of white blood cells called natural killer (NK) cells. Of all the immune systems cells, NK cells have shown the strongest links to fighting cancer, specifically preventing metastasis and destroying small metastases. Although the result of this study is not definitive, it indicates that stress acts by suppressing NK-cell activity.

Another 1999 study [Stone AA, Mezzacappa ES, Donatone BA, Gonder M. Psychosocial stress and social support are associated with prostate-specific antigen in men: Results from a community screening program. Health Psychology. 1999;18:482–486] showed stress and social support are important influences in a man's risk of developing prostate cancer. Researchers at State University of New York at Stony Brook's medical school found men with high levels of stress and a lack of satisfying relationships with friends and family had higher levels of Prostate-Specific Antigen (PSA) in their blood, a marker for an increased risk of developing prostate cancer.

Based on the results, the risk of having an abnormal PSA was three times higher for men with high levels of stress. Likewise, men who had felt they had low levels of support from friends and family were twice as likely to have an abnormal PSA. The findings strongly indicate (or "possibly suggest" if you are a non-believer) that a man's psychological state can have a direct impact on prostate disease.

PSYCHONEUROIMMUNOLOGY (PNI)

The study of the physical effects of the mind on the immune system is called psychoneuroimmunology. Why is that important? Because cancer is very much an issue with the immune system.

In our current understanding of "The Emperor Of All Maladies", as cancer has been called, we all throw out cancer cells all the time. There are some in everyone's blood, at any one time. But the immune system can spot the rogue cells and eliminate them. Supporting your immune system is therefore of paramount importance in avoiding or recovering from cancer.

The most important cells in the immune system for fighting cancer are the natural killer (NK) cells. NK cells were discovered 40 years ago, by their ability to recognize and kill tumor cells without the requirement of prior antigen exposure. Since then, NK cells have been seen as promising agents for cell-based cancer therapies. Disappointingly, only limited anti-tumor effects have been demonstrated following NK cell transplant (infusion) in patients with solid tumors. While NK cells have great potential in targeting tumor cells in circulation, the efficiency of NK cell activity right inside the tumor is yet unclear.

[Natural Killer Cell-Based Therapies Targeting Cancer: Possible Strategies to Gain and Sustain Anti-Tumor Activity. *Front Immunol.* 2015; 6: 605. doi: 10.3389/fimmu.2015.00605

The idea that NK cells patrol the body, eliminating cancer cells as they develop, is called the "immune surveillance theory". One of the early proponents of immune surveillance and the man who coined the term psychoneuroimmunology, Nobel Laureate Dr. F. Macfarlane Burnet, pointed out that a weak immune system can make people more susceptible to cancer. The frequency of Kaposi's sarcoma among AIDS patients is an example of a cancer developing when the immune system is damaged. [Burnet FM. Cancer – A biological approach. 1. The process of control. Br Med J. 1957;1:779–782]

Chronic depression has been identified as an element in the development of cancer. We also know that depression can lower our immune function. Is this beginning to hang together for you?

An investigation of the relationship between depression and cancer called the Chicago Study followed two thousand workers at Western Electric for seventeen years. The researchers found that those who had significant depression on the Minnesota Multiphasic Personality Inventory (MMPI) scale were 2.5 times more likely to develop cancer later in life. [Personality and risk of cancer: 20-year follow-up of the Western Electric Study. *Psychosom Med.* 1987 Sep-Oct;49(5):435-49].

Spontaneous Remission

More evidence for PNI comes from the spontaneous remission of established cancers. In a study of 130 clear cases of spontaneous remission of malignant tumors, the only explanation for these cases seems to be that the immune system seemed to come alive and learn to recognize the cancer cells and destroy them. The mind is very capable of initiating this process (but only by removing the negative factors that brought about trouble in the first place).

Cancer Ward

Internationally-acclaimed oncologist (now retired) Bernie Siegel MD suggests the term "creative or self-induced healing," or "hard work miracle," rather than spontaneous healing. Russian novelist Aleksandr Solzhenitsyn wrote of self-induced healing in *Cancer Ward* (Farrar, Straus, Giroux, 1969):

Kostoglotov...[said]..."we shouldn't behave like rabbits and put our complete trust in doctors. For instance, I'm reading this book." He picked up a large, open book from the window sill. "Abrikososov and Stryukov, Pathological Anatomy, medical school textbook. It says here that the link between the development of tumors and the central nervous system has so far been very little studied. And this link is an amazing thing! It's written here in so many words." He found the place. "It happens rarely, but there are cases of self-induced healing. You see how it's worded? Not recovery through treatment, but actual healing. See?"

There was a stir throughout the ward. It was as though "self-induced healing" had fluttered out of the great open book like a rainbow-colored butterfly for everyone to see, and they all held up their foreheads and cheeks for its healing touch as it flew past.

"Self-induced," said Kostoglotov, laying aside his book. He waved his hands, fingers splayed. ... "That means that suddenly for some unexplained reason the tumor starts off in the opposite direction! It gets smaller, resolves and finally disappears! See?"

They were all silent, gaping at the fairy tale. That a tumor, one's own tumor, the destructive tumor which had mangled one's whole life, should suddenly drain away, dry up and die by itself?

They were all silent, still holding their faces up to the butterfly. It was only the gloomy Podduyev who made his bed creak and, with a hopeless and obstinate expression on his face, croaked out, "I suppose for that you need to have...a clear conscience."

Note that spontaneous remission is a word used by orthodox doctors to cover up the fact that:

a) They really don't understand why the patient recovered

b) They don't recognize nature's ability to bring about healing without intervention from a physician.

So it must be "spontaneous", whatever that means.

Spontaneous remission, as it is often referred to, caught the attention of Kelly Turner, PhD, when she was an undergraduate at Harvard University in Boston. "I was surprised how little research was being done by the medical community on these patients who had healed from cancer," she said in an interview for Medscape. "Many of the patients had healed without undergoing Western medical treatment or, following its failure, they used other therapies to extend their survival." [http://www.medscape.com/viewarticle/827945]

Turner came across her first case of radical remission when she was working as a counselor at a major cancer center. Intrigued, she conducted a quick search of the medical literature and was surprised to find there were over 1000 cases reported in medical journals, and counting.

These were primarily case studies, but there was no information about how the patient managed to survive. "No one had asked the patients what they had done to heal," Dr. Turner explained.

It became the focus of her PhD thesis at the University of California, Berkeley. Dr. Turner's research involved a year-long trip to 10 countries to interview 50 holistic healers and scores of cancer survivors about healing techniques. Since that time, she has analyzed more than 1000 cases of spontaneous remission and written a book: *Radical Remission: Surviving Cancer Against All Odds*. Of the cases that she reviewed, about 85% have no evidence of disease on their medical charts. About 15% still have cancer, but their tumors have shrunk and have remained stable for years.

Dr. Turner prefers the term "radical remission" because typically there is nothing spontaneous about these unusual cures. Most patients were actively doing something to facilitate healing.

9 healing factors stood out, of which 5 may be said to be mental/psychological:
1. releasing suppressed emotions
2. increasing positive emotions
3. embracing social support
4. deepening spiritual connection
5. having a strong reasons for living

[http://www.medscape.com/viewarticle/827945#vp_1]

In 1993, the Institute of Noetic Sciences published *Spontaneous Remissions: An Annotated Bibliography*, which catalogued the world's medical literature on the subject. It included references to cancer and a wide range of illnesses — from ulcers to injuries caused by gunshots. It is essentially the largest database of medically reported cases of spontaneous remission in the world, with more than 3500 references from more than 800 journals in 20 languages.

Some research in this area has been conducted by Moshe Frenkel, MD, from Integrative Oncology Consultants, who is a clinical associate professor at the University of Texas Medical Branch in Galveston.

"The issue of exceptional patients has been an interest of mine for over 20 years. I have met hundreds of patients that fit the criteria in the medical arena," he told Medscape Medical News.

In one study of 14 medically exceptional outcomes, Dr. Frenkel and colleagues found that the overarching theme was connections, both internal and external [Palliat Support Care. 2013:1-8]. Internal connections include relationships with God or a higher power and with oneself. The external connections include relationships with friends and family, with the medical system (physician, nurses, and other staff), and with other patients.

THE IMMUNE CONNECTION

Several pathways showing that the brain and nervous system affect the immune system have been discovered. Most of the brain/immune-system connections relate to ways of coping with stress. With sudden stress the brain stimulates the adrenal glands to release adrenaline and other powerful stress response hormones. We call this the hypothalamic-pituitary-adrenal axis. Unfortunately, this response dampens the immune response.

Under chronic stress the adrenal gland puts out a critical hormone, called cortisol, which suppresses the immune system, especially the NK cells that attack cancer. When mice prone to developing breast cancer were repeatedly stressed with foot shocks, they had reduced NK cell activity and shortened survival time.

In fact the best illustration I know of the damaging effects of cortisol is the story of the annual Pacific salmon run. Millions of fish struggle upstream in what are immensely stressful challenges, against often ferocious currents. Usually they make it and spawn successfully. But few fish ever make it back to the ocean. Almost at once the salmon waste away and quickly die off, being consumed by bacteria and fungus. They look terrible, almost rotting while still alive! But what you may not know is that the cortisol levels in the salmon are up to 3,000 times the normal amount. As a consequence have they have virtually no immunity to fight off infections.

IS THERE A CANCER-PRONE PERSONALITY TYPE?

Health workers have been asking this question for decades. There is still plenty of debate. We know that emotions such as depression, anger, and hostility make us more prone to illness and disease; and it's been shown that positive attitudes such as hope, optimism, and happiness strengthens our immune system and protects us from disease.

So why are we even asking if character traits and mental make-up are an influence in health and diseases such as cancer?

I already mentioned the Roman/Greek physician Galen believed that melancholy (depression) makes an individual more prone to cancer. It's a theme that has cycled around and around since that time.

There may in fact be two types of personality, making us either cancer-prone or cancer resistant.

The cancer-prone type can be quickly summed up as:
•   Represses emotions (both positive and negative).
•   Shows anger, resentment, or hostility towards others.
•   Takes on extra duties and responsibilities, even when they cause stress.
•   Reacts adversely to and does not cope well with life changes.
•   Is negative or pessimistic.
•   Becomes easily depressed or has feelings of hopelessness.
•   Worries often and excessively about others.
•   Feels the need for approval and to please others.

As professor Andrew Goliszek at North Carolina A&T State University points out, there are always exceptions: some of the most optimistic and positive among us will get cancer, and some of the angriest and most hostile will live to be 100, cancer-free. But when a cancer patient is told that his or her disease is terminal, those who adopt cancer-resistant traits tend to live longer because their newly acquired behaviors will automatically boost immunity.

Cancer-Resistant Personality Type
- Expresses emotions in a positive and constructive way.
- Controls anger and resolves anger issues positively.
- Knows when to say no.
- Copes well with stress and feels in control of situations.
- Is optimistic and hopeful.
- Does not become easily depressed.
- Seeks out and maintains social support networks.
- Does not worry excessively.
- Likes to please, but does not seek approval as an emotional crutch.

The Type C Personality

Researchers from Johns Hopkins University began a long term prospective study, starting in 1946, to see if psychological factors could predict future disease states. They followed 1,130 medical students over 18 years. The results came as a surprise to them.

"Our results appear to agree with findings that cancer patients 'tend to deny and repress conflictual impulses and emotions to a higher degree than do other people.'"

Studies in the 1940s and 1950s continued to explore this idea but it wasn't until 1979 that the "Type C personality" (C for cancer) was coined by Dr. Lydia Temoshok, Director of The Behavioral Medicine Program, Biotechnology Institute, University of Maryland Medical School.

What Dr. Temoshok found in interviewing 150 melanoma patients was a striking and amazingly similar pattern of behaviors. These patients were overwhelmingly nice. Yes, they were excessively nice, pleasant to a fault, uncomplaining and unassertive. They went far out of their way and changed their schedules to make time to talk with her—so as not to disappoint her. They seemed extremely worried about their disease progression--but not for themselves. They worried about the effect it was having on their families: "I'm fine, but I'm really worried about my husband. He takes things so hard..."

In effect, they were in a form of denial and using it as a coping strategy. Temoshok began to suspect that there was much more than simple denial at work and she soon began to recognize a common pattern. These patients were "pleasers" who had spent their entire lives trying to be accepted by others—spouses, parents, siblings, coworkers, friends etc. In fact, their very identities seemed to be derived from how they were perceived by others in their lives.

Temoshok describes this as "Out of touch with their primary needs and emotions, they look to others for signals on how to think, feel and act." She named this set of behavior traits and coping methods the "Type C" phenomenon and she developed her theories from psychological, social and biological perspectives.

According to Temoshok, "....What they shared was a manner of handling life stress. The melanoma patients coped by keeping their feelings under wraps. They never expressed anger, and rarely did they acknowledge fear and sadness. They maintained a façade of pleasantness even under the most painful or aggravating circumstances. They strived excessively to please people they cared about, to please authority figures, even to please strangers."

Since that time, other physicians have been able to confirm this finding in a clinical setting.

Canadian homeopathic doctor Alexander Mostovoy adds a few more Type C traits...

- They are more likely to grieve or worry unduly over a personal loss. This could be a financial loss or loss of status as well as loss of a loved one.

- They have a passion that has remained unfulfilled and suppressed over many years.

- They feel unworthy. They put others' needs before themselves. They tend to be really nice people.

- They avoid conflict or arguments, can't express hostility, are punctual, neat and tidy, always strive for perfection, work too hard, overachieve and find it difficult to relax.

For over half a century the late Dr. W. Douglas Brodie, founder of the Reno Integrative Medical Center in Nevada and a pioneer of integrative treatments for cancer, found that there were consistent personality traits among the many thousands of his cancer patients.

In addition to the attributes already described, Dr. Brodie found his patients often were not close to one or both parents. This may have been a problem early in their lives or occurred later in life. He believed it was linked to a lack of intimacy with their spouse or family member.

In his work as a psychologist in a New York City cancer hospital for over 30 years, Dr. Lawrence LeShan observed another thread amongst cancer patients, which was an unfulfilled passion that had been suppressed for many years. For example, a child who wanted to learn the piano, but couldn't because either their parents could not afford those piano lessons, or other priorities took precedence over theirs.

This pattern of suppression would repeat itself over their lifetime. Oddly enough, studying piano later in life, or fulfilling a previously unfulfilled passion has an amazing curative effect.

Of course there are always researchers who debunk things. It's fashionable just now to deny the effects of personality on contracting any disease, including cancer. Remember this is the view that the pharmaceutical industry wants carried forward (wink wink!)

A review of studies in 2010 concluded that they "do not give much support to personality as a causative factor for cancer." [Future Oncol. 2010 May;6(5):691-707. doi: 10.2217/fon.10.31.]

Another review in 2014 included over 42,000 people and more than 2,000 suffering from six types of cancer amongst them. They looked at five personality traits – extraversion (sociable, outgoing personality), neuroticism, agreeableness, conscientiousness, and openness to experience.

They concluded that "none of the personality traits were associated with the incidence of all cancers or any of the six site-specific cancers." [http://www.ncbi.nlm.nih.gov/pubmed/24504367]

It may be true that personality is not such a big causative factor in the development of all cancers. More important perhaps are smoking, alcohol consumption, excessive dietary sugars (and other carbs), nutrient-poor diets, poor exercise habits, poor sleep habits and exposure to toxins, to name a key few.

But it makes sense to deal with what you CAN deal with. Just as people may change their diet, cut out smoking or reduce their environmental exposure to toxins in order to lower their cancer risk, so you should try to address negative aspects of your personality that may be impacting health. Getting stress out of your life is essential not only to avoiding cancer, but to happiness in general.

STRESS IS THE KILLER

Stress is different. It does not relate to personality traits. It relates to our environment or—more exactly—our response to the environment. It's particularly difficult to define, since stressful influences vary from one individual to another. One person could find a demanding job extremely stressful, while another would enjoy the challenge. What is restful calm to one person may be unendurable boredom to another.

I have an amazingly good and useful definition of stress: *stress is the difference between what you have and what you wanted*. Think about that... the wider the gap between the two—the more the disconnect between your desires and your circumstances—the more stress you will feel.

Another definition of stressful influences can be *those events or activities that exceed the individual's ability to cope comfortably*. Stress is perhaps the ultimate subjective variable, and the best way to be sure an event is stressful is to ask the person himself.

Stress has a strong effect on the development and outcome of cancer. It has been shown that there is a correlation between stressful life events such as the death of a family member or the breakdown of important family relationships and relapse of breast cancer.

Hamer's Controversy

No text of this kind would be complete without visiting the controversy raging around Dr. Reike Geerd Hamer's work. He has his followers who virtually worship him and call his "German New Medicine" "La Medicine Sagrada" (sacred medicine). But critics abound and are relentlessly vicious.

The Swiss Cancer League described Hamer's approach as "dangerous, especially as it lulls the patients into a false sense of security, so that they are deprived of other effective treatments." Of course when you think through what they mean by "effective treatments", you know at once they are not to be trusted.

The picture internationally is one of suppression and misrepresentation. What was all the fuss? He came up with a extensive theory about how and why emotional shocks could lead to disease, particularly cancer (more details in a moment).

Perhaps the real key to the storm which has raged for decades is that Hamer, perhaps unthinkingly, criticized a member of the European royalty. Let me tell you the story in brief, and see what you think!

Hamer, a German doctor with his own practice in Rome, received a call in the middle of the night saying his 17-year old son Dirk had been shot by an Italian prince of the House of Savoy, while he was asleep on a boat anchored on the island of Cavallo. It was said to be an accidental shooting; there were no witnesses; the Prince was never charged with any crime. Three months later, Dirk died.

Not long afterwards, Hamer—who had been healthy all his life—found he had testicular cancer. He put two and two together and realized that the psychic trauma of his son's death had probably precipitated the cancer.

The question was: would that apply generally to cancer patients? Hamer set about doing research on the personal histories of cancer patients to see whether they had suffered some shock, distress or trauma before their illness.

In time, after extensive research on some 31,000 patients, Hamer concluded that disease (not just cancer) is brought about by a shock for which we are totally unprepared, that a physical event can create a biological conflict shock that manifests in a visible physical transformation in the brain, and leads to a measurable change in physical-neurological parameters and to the development of cancerous growths, ulcerations, necroses and functional disturbances in specific organs of the body.

Hamer calls this the "iron rule" of cancer. In typical Germanic fashion, he claimed this was an absolute law: no exceptions. That may be whimsy. But he was certainly onto something.

In fact Hamer has laid out five separate "biological laws". He realized that "diseases" were not meaningless mistakes of nature that should be fought with frenzy, but meaningful events that serve to heal and restore equilibrium. I'm totally with him on that one [see also *The Healing Power Of Disease*, by Thorwald Dethlefsen and Dr. Rudiger Dahlke, Vega, 2002]. German-born Thorwald Dethlefsen is probably best known as a spiritual psychologist.

The shock element is critical and affects mind, brain and body. But if we can in any way be prepared for the shocking event, we will not become ill, says Hamer. More importantly, if we can effectively UN-do the shock, recovery can take place, actually rather easily. In fact, Dr. Hamer does not like to say 'cancer'. Rather, it is a special biological response to an unusual situation, and when the 'shock' situation is resolved, the body sets about returning to normality.

His "5 Laws" are otherwise as follows:

1. Every disease is caused by a conflict shock that catches an individual completely off guard.

2. Provided there is a resolution of the conflict, every disease proceeds in two phases, a conflict-active phase and a healing phase.

3. This law ties the findings of the first two laws into the context of embry-ology and the evolution of man. It illustrates the biological correlation between the psyche, the brain, and the organ from an evolutionary point of view. (The Ontogenetic System of Tumors and Cancer-Equivalent Diseases)

4. Addresses the role of microbes in the context of evolution and in rela-tion to the three germ layers from which our organs originate. Microbes are indispensable to your survival.

5. Every so-called disease has to be understood as a "meaningful special biological program of nature" created to solve an unexpected biological conflict.

Laws 1 and 2 led Hamer to frame a model of cancer as a healing process: there is a starting conflict-active stage, precipitating the disease process, which he named the Dirk Hamer Syndrome in honor of his son (not a good choice, in my view; this must have irked the Prince's powerful and well-con-nected family).

The initial stage is followed by a healing stage, in which disturbances are resolved, the disease process is cleaned up by natural processes and nor-mality returns.

Even more controversially, Hamer believes that a person cannot die of can-cer in and of itself.

If someone dies during the conflict-active phase of disease, he says, it's because of energy loss, weight loss, sleep deprivation, and emotional and mental exhaustion. The stress of receiving a cancer diagnosis, or being given a negative prognosis, is often enough to deprive a person of their life-force. Conventional cancer treatments only accelerate the downward spiral.

Well, to attack the Cancer Mafia is a good way to find yourself attacked, isolated and even criminalized, and that's exactly what happened.

The hostility to which Hamer has been subjected since publishing his findings is even worse than the usual onslaughts from conventional medicine. His license to practise medicine was withdrawn (which remains true to this day).

He took the University of Tubingen to court and won; the University was ordered by the court to hold tests to verify Hamer's theories. They have never done so. Instead they launched vicious personal assaults, media campaigns, investigations and even criminal attempts to have him forcibly committed to a psychiatric institution (you can imagine what kind of "treatment" he would have received in there). Hamer was even jailed for 18 months on the pretext of illegally practising medicine, when he offered information to patients about his "New Medicine".

Like many of us, Hamer believes very strongly that the present methods of dealing with cancer are barbarous, cruel and completely unnecessary. This opinion does not make him many friends among those who actually carry out these destructive treatments.

However it should be pointed out that a great deal of the opposition Hamer has faced allegedly come from the very man who killed his son, the Prince of Savoy, son of the last King of Italy. It would be impossible to say, without intervention from the CIA and Interpol, which simply isn't going to happen.

The controversy still prevents many cancer sufferers from getting to grips with his work. You can Google this story. But beware: *there is no official Hamer website!* I can recommend Caroline Markolin's site, because I have studied Hamer's materials with her and know that he considers her his mouthpiece. The two exchange views regularly. [http://www.germannewmedicine.ca/home.html]

Other websites are mostly self-serving advertizing platforms.

Markolin's group hosts an annual International GNM Conference, which over the years has been attended by participants from 32 nations, including Australia, New Zealand, China, India, Russia, South Africa, the United States, Canada, and Mexico as well as most countries in South America and Europe. Many of her students are now teaching the GNM principles in their own right.

I fully support Markolin's teaching platform.

And it will be no surprise to know that many other workers have expressed the same or similar views as Hamer. It makes you wonder why there is such a strong kickback against obvious basic principles. Is it jealousy among colleagues? Was Hamer so abrasive that he naturally created enmity? (it happens; in fact it happens a lot) Or just royalty abusing their powers?

One study group is interesting to note, in that they actually quantified the effects of stress (twice actually) and the results may surprise you...

The Life Events Scale

Probably the most famous analysis of the health consequences of stress is the so-called Holmes-Rahe Social Readjustment Rating Scale (1977). Thomas H. Holmes and Richard H. Rahe of the University of Washington School of Medicine interviewed over 5,000 cases and showed that the more stress you experienced, the more likely it was that you would suffer some kind of health breakdown in the subsequent 2 years.

They went further and were able to produce a league table of disaster, which rated each life event according to severity and likeliness of ill-health. The top 3 events concern break up of longstanding relationships, whether by death or divorce and this will come as no surprise to those who have had to endure such suffering. Also appearing are marriage, change of job, jail term, pregnancy and large mortgage. It is interesting to note that even what are supposed to be pleasing life events, nevertheless carry their stress toll (marriage, birth and getting a raise).

A new scale of rankings were drawn up in 1997 by US psychiatrists from the Veterans Affairs Medical Centre in Reno, Nevada, based on a study of 427 volunteers who were asked to assess 87 life events.

The study was published in the *Journal of Psychosomatic Research* and reported by *Hospital Doctor*. Women scored 86 of the 87 events as more stressful men. But, so the explanation goes, it is not women who are over-reacting but men who are under-reacting!

It was reckoned that stress, overall, has increased by 45% in the 40-year period since the first study was conducted.

Unmarried people gave higher scores across the range of events. It suggests that being married or attached is a far safer way to face life's trials and that you will live longer and be more healthy if you are married. This has been shown before to be a true medical fact.

The top 15 stressors on both old and new scales are as follows:

1977.	1997.
1. Death of spouse	1. Death of spouse
2. Death of close family member	2. Divorce
3. Fired from work	3. Death of close family member
4. Divorce	4. Marital separation
5. Pregnancy	5. Fired from work
6. Jail term	6. Major illness or injury
7. Loan repayment demand	7. Jail term
8. Marital separation	8. Death of close friend
9. Change in health of family member	9. Pregnancy
10. Marriage	10. Major business readjustment
11. Retirement	11. Loan repayment demand
12. Sexual difficulties	12. Gain new family member
13. Change in financial state	13. Marital reconciliation
14. Gain new family member	14. Change in health of family member
15. Death of close friend	15. Change in financial state

Natural Killer Cells and Stress

An ever-increasing number of studies are showing that stress and depression suppress NK cell activity. In a seminal study conducted at the University of Rochester in New York State by Robert Ader, professor of psychiatry and psychology, rats were given cyclophosphamide, a powerful form of chemotherapy, in a saccharine solution. Cyclophosphamide causes unpleasant stomach pain. It was no surprise that soon the rats associated the sweetened water with the pain and refused to drink it.

Strangely, at a later date, when the rats were given saccharine alone, they started dying off simply because their immune systems were conditioned to associate the sweet taste of harmless saccharine with the poisonous chemotherapy.

Cyclophosphamide, in addition to causing stomach discomfort, suppresses the immune system. More experiments confirmed that tasting the saccharine alone triggered the nervous system to suppress the immune system.

It was the start of psychoneuroimmunology. Prior to this work, no connection between the mind and the immune system was thought to exist.

"Today there is not a physician in the country who does not accept the science Bob Ader set in motion," said Dr. Bruce Rabin, founder of the Brain, Behavior and Immunity Center at the University of Pittsburgh Medical Center, who considered Dr. Ader a mentor. "He attracted interest in the field and made it possible to prove that 'mind-body' is real." [NY Times obituary, Dec 25, 2011: http://www.nytimes.com/2011/12/26/science/robert-ader-who-linked-stress-and-illness-dies-at-79.html?_r=2&ref=obituaries]

Sandra Levy and others investigated the correlation between NK cell activity and mood. Levy found that healthy people who felt they were under stress had persistently low NK cell activity. In a study of cancer patients she found that NK cell activity was not affected by chemotherapy or radiotherapy, but was correlated with three indicators of distress: patient adjustment, lack of social support, and symptoms of fatigue and depression. [Correlation of stress factors with sustained depression of natural killer cell activity and predicted prognosis in patients with breast cancer. S Levy, R Herberman, M Lippman and T d'Angelo; *Journal of Clinical Oncology*, March 1, 1987: 348-353]

Michael Irwin has carried out several studies of links between NK cell activity and depression. His research team found that women whose husbands had recently died showed reduced NK cell activity. [Depression and reduced natural killer cytotoxicity: a longitudinal study of depressed patients and control subjects, *Psychological Medicine*, Volume 22, Issue 4, November 1992, pp. 1045-1050]

These studies clearly demonstrate that our emotions and moods can affect the immune system. We also know that a healthy immune system is essential to disease prevention. But does the state of the immune system extend to preventing and controlling cancer?

Cancer may bring on a range of emotions, including, but not limited to, the following:

- Shock/disbelief
- Fear/uncertainty
- Guilt
- Grief/sadness
- Anxiety
- Depression
- Anger/frustration
- Feelings of isolation
- Vulnerability/helplessness

As I remarked earlier, cancer itself is a *huge* stress. Survivors can develop PTSD. One study published in 2011 in the *Journal of Clinical Oncology* found that more than one-third of the 566 Non-Hodgkin's lymphoma survivors the researchers tracked for PTSD reported chronic or worsened symptoms over the course of five years. The research team concluded that health care providers should be vigilant for PTSD in their patients with cancer to increase the odds of staving it off and connecting patients with appropriate mental health treatment.

OCYTOCIN TO THE RESCUE

My friend Norman Shealy MD, founder of the American Holistic Medical Association, has developed a wonderful healing and calming model, guaranteed to raise your HRV (page 88)!

It's called the Ring Of Air, a series of 13 acupuncture points which—when stimulated—releases oxytocin, the soothing "love hormone".

New research is suggesting that oxytocin plays a crucial part in enabling us not just to forge and strengthen our social relations, but in helping us to stave off a number of psychological and physiological problems as well.

One of the nice things about oxytocin is that you can get your fix anywhere and at any time. All you need to do is simply hug someone, kiss or just shake their hand! The simple act of bodily contact will cause your brain to release low levels of oxytocin—both in yourself and in the person you're touching. It's a near-instantaneous way to establish trust. And the good news is that the effect lingers afterward.

And you shouldn't feel limited to people; it also helps to hug and play with animals.

You can take extra oxytocin as a spray. It works, but it doesn't last. You need to take it four times a day. A better plan is to persuade your body to make its own oxytocin...

The Ring Of Air

This is where Norman Shealy's marvelous improvement comes into its own. By stimulating the so-called "Ring Of Air", we can get the body to release its own oxytocin. Originally this was researched using electrical acupuncture stimulation, but Norman's *even better* idea is using a proprietary blend of essential oils, called Air Bliss.

It works from a roll-on applicator. The great thing about the applicator model is that you don't have to be spot-on accurate. The result is relaxation and happiness, after about 30 minutes. Norm jokes he's been asked, "Is this stuff legal?" and told "This has street value, Doc!"

The acupuncture points to use are these, starting at the bottom and working up to the skull crown:
- Spleen 1A, bilaterally
- Liver 3, bilaterally
- Stomach 36, bilaterally
- Governing Vessel 1, 16 and 20
- Gall Bladder 20, bilaterally
- Lung 1, bilaterally

You can use a reference book to work out where these points are. Or you can watch a video of Norman applying Air Bliss to these points on a volunteer subject (see below).

Why Oxytocin?

Oxytocin is known as a hormone for "forgetting one's self"; it is also known as the "bliss hormone". When you have plenty, life does indeed seem charmed and blessed.

Life events which can lower or even block oxytocin include PTSD, depression, anxiety, childhood trauma and certain cases of autism. [G Missig, et al. Oxytocin Reduces Background Anxiety in a Fear-Potentiated Startle Paradigm. *Neuropsychopharmacology*. 2010; 35: 2607–2616]

Oxytocin, not surprisingly then, helps relieve depression and anxiety. It naturally enhances a sense of:
- Optimism
- Trust
- Mastery
- Self-esteem

These are very powerful feelings for sufferers with cancer.

Studies have also shown that a rise in oxytocin levels can relieve pain, which could be useful to some patients. The hard part is getting up your oxytocin levels while feeling the pain. That's where sprays can help.

Best of all is Norman's simple-to-use Air Bliss applied correctly.

You can obtain supplies easly, online, from normshealy.com [https://normshealy.com/the-sacred-rings/the-ring-of-air/] and there you can watch a video of how to apply it.

Note: Air Bliss has been shown to raise levels of Neurotensin, too, for natural pain relief.

PART 2
HOW WE CAN COMBAT IT

Cancer Is A Career Change.

You are facing danger. Elsewhere I have written that battling cancer needs to be a career change. You cannot afford to leave it to the doctor and just hope for the best.

It bears repeating: cancer is a wake up call but it is not a death knell. It tells you loud and clear that something is wrong with your life and lifestyle and that has now reduced your health and vitality to ruinous levels. You must listen to the message from Mother Nature and take appropriate action.

If you heed the warnings, and correct your erroneous ways, you will be quite safe. Many people have had cause to bless the fact that they got cancer: it alerted them to the fact that their life was wildly off track and that they must do something effective to put matters right—or pay the ultimate price.

My other books, especially *Cancer Research Secrets*, will tell you what your treatment alternatives are. You'll be surprised how many different actions you can take that will raise your chances of beating the disease successfully. In fact I'd like to encourage you that, in the early stages at least, cancer isn't that difficult to conquer at all.

Doctors insist on making stupid prognostications. These are often wrong. But in any case, they may become a self-fulfilling prophecy. The patient's subconscious will take this pronouncement on board and make it come true. That way the doctor looks good – he or she got it right. But it doesn't come under the role of a doctor, as I understand the term role.

The fact is that every disease you can name, of every severity, has been survived by others before you. People sick unto death and not expected to last the day have got up and walked out of hospital; terminal cancer patients, whose bodies were riddled with secondaries, have recovered and the tumors gone away (and stayed away for the rest of their lives); people who were paralyzed have walked again (done a few of those myself) and even genetically- determined conditions have disappeared, no matter the DNA message.

You will come to the fascinating and inspiring story of Anita Moorjani in a later section (page 109).

The fact is, whatever you are facing, there is a path back to health. You may have been living where this path is very hidden and overgrown with intellectual weeds. But it's there. It's ALWAYS there. You only have to find your path!

I repeat the obvious: To beat cancer you must take charge of your own health. You need to become the executive manager or chief-of-staff for your own case. Don't be panicked by threats that you will die horribly and quickly if you do not opt for surgery, chemo or radiation: doctors who treat you in this way are a disgrace to the profession and should lose their right to practice. Remember their motivation is primarily to make money from your plight; platitudes and assurances are really only to disguise the financial nature of their interests.

At the same time, I am not saying that you must necessarily abandon the conventional approach. The final choice must be yours and not some oncologist panting for the cash for a down payment on his or her second or third home. Unfortunately, in some territories (such as here in California), it is illegal for a doctor to offer any other therapy than conventional chemo or radiation. That's "freedom" for you.

Notwithstanding the political failings of these crazy bureaucracies, there is thankfully no law that says you must abide by what the oncologist recommends. For the time being, at least, even Californians have the right to opt out of the mainstream approach (some of us are concerned that even this small freedom will eventually be taken away).

But you must then take over and act. That includes a whole shift in attitude and belief systems. You won't get well accepting the indoctrination that you cannot get well. Just remember that!

MEETING WITH A FEISTY LUNG CANCER SURVIVOR

In 2014, while visiting Scotland, I was privileged to meet someone very special. For anonymity, let's call her Tash, which is her nickname. She was a lady who had survived small-cell carcinoma of the lung and was coming up to the 5-year mark. This is a deadly tumor. Not many people make it to the 5-year point (less than 10%).

Having read one of her letters to her consultant specialist, which was brimming with fire, scorn, irony and wit, I decided she was someone I needed to meet. What was her survival secret?

I already knew part of it: a blatant contempt for science, statistics (especially) and doctors with a dire attitude! You have read my comments on this before: those patients who do best with cancer are not the meek and obedient ones but the ones with a feisty "Go f**k yourself" sort attitude to the medical profession.

Tash describes herself as a "bolshie old fart". It could be life-saving, as we Boomers know.

So, one fine sunny day (it later turned to torrential rain) I made my way to the town of Gairloch, in the beautiful Western Highlands of Scotland and met Tash. My wife Vivien was with me.

The lady was gracious but at once lively and entertaining, with not a hint of gloom; quips seem to be as natural to her as breathing. Not surprising, since she describes herself as a columnist, poet and political cartoonist. We sat down over tea and I listened to the story, starting with my question "Tell us about who and what you are?"

Like me, she had grown up in the 1960s "flower power" era; she was at that time a well-known person in the Scottish folk music scene. This was also the time of free love and the result was a child which, under pressure, she had had adopted. For completeness, it should be said that, at age 30, he found his Mum and has forgiven her completely. He turned too out to be an artist and a musician.

Eventually forced to face the economic realities of life (grow up, in other words), Tash had graduated at university and gone to work as a civil servant in the Scottish Office. That career lasted decades until, on a wild impulse, ad quit her job and gone to Australia. Likely she would still be there, she confided in me, but that her father fell fatally ill and she came back to Scotland.

From there came a period of uncertainty, leading up to the diagnosis. As I always do, I asked for the episode of real stress that preceded the illness (I agree with Dr. Ryke Geerd Hamer page 22 there is almost always a prior psychic trauma). There was no doubt in Tash's case...

She had moved to a small town where things were pretty rough (Aultbea). The local louts had taken it on themselves to run a hate campaign against her and made life intolerable. There were threats of violence and she genuinely feared for her safety; so much so that, as well as locking and double locking the door, she habitually wedged a chair against the letterbox, so that nothing harmful could be pushed through it at night.

Tash eventually fled the town and settled in Gairloch, but the damage was done. It started as a persistent cough and then one day there was blood. In someone who had smoked heavily, even though she had given up for many years, it was bad news...

So came the grim diagnosis of small-cell cancer of the lung. Tash accepted the recommendation for chemo and radiotherapy but wisely decided to try and throw other treatment modalities at it.

"No, I'm not having this!" she raged to herself and others. Interestingly she explained to me that she came to think of her cancer as the "Aultbea disease" and that with this tumor she was "getting rid of Aultbea." This incredible insight shows that she was wise beyond her doctors. Cancer is often an expression of something that needs to heal. Ah, if only the majority doctors new that...

Well, heal she did. Within four months, this deadly tumor was gone from her body.

Coincidentally, she had a friend in Edinburgh diagnosed with small-cell lung cancer at about the same time. That friend is now dead. The difference is hardly down to lousy doctoring; the difference was that the friend accepted her doom, just as the doctors pronounced it. She didn't even want to talk about it, while in contrast Tash took the rise out of doctors and talked about her cancer to everybody.

So what was her strategy? What did she do? Stay away from pessimists was one keynote (she later found her friends were very pessimistic but had managed to hide it). She had her lucky stones; I saw them but wasn't allowed to touch. There was a snowflake obsidian, the cancer stone; jasper for courage; and she showed me what she called a recovery stone, to be sure it wasn't coming back. She also tried homeopathy, a remedy called *mulla mulla* from Australia (it's a remedy for fire and she took it during the "fire" of radiation therapy).

She had people praying for her, even though she is dismissive of organized religions. "The purpose of life is living", is her motto. There was a church in Africa that sang and prayed for her. A Buddhist in Nairn offered to pray for her. A lady in the spiritual church in Livingstone also asked and Mary, the mother of a friend at the Roman Catholic church in Edinburgh. "For all I know it could be Mary that cured me," she quipped.

There was also the feeling of a lot of support from my friends; "a network of love" as she described it. I'm covering a lot of this throughout the book.

The key thing in her case was the use of internal imaging, "visualization" as it's called. Sometimes it's good to nurture your cancer cells; talk to them nicely and try to persuade them home to health. But none of that for Tash; she wanted them dead, D-E-A-D! Gone!

Being a country-based person, for that she enlisted the aid of imaginary sheep dogs. As she explained to me, there was a need to stop the rogue cells escaping control, to prevent them running amok and metastasizing. What does rounding things up and keeping them penned in bring to mind? Obviously, sheep dogs. She used two: a mother, Meg, and her son Rob.

For those of you who like woo-woo (Celtic Scotland is oozing with woo-stuff), a friend took a picture of two nice sheepdogs she saw in the back of a truck one day, for no reason apparently, and got the thought she should send the photo to Tash, again for no logical reason. The friend did not know about the visualizations. But when she got the gift, Tash recognized the dogs in the photograph as exact look-alikes of her imaginary Meg and Rob.

They had warned Tash that radiotherapy could burn her gullet and throw her appetite off. When asked how she coped, Tash humorously told the doctors, "I can't tolerate the more robust New World reds any more!" (translation: rich, flavorsome red wines from California and Australia).

Fortunately, she had now got over this "disability"! So, as if on cue, I sent Vivien out for a nice, smooth, full-bodied New World shiraz, which we all enjoyed together lustily as we continued to talk.

When it came to the radiotherapy, she had adopted a different visualization, which was a countryman, with wellington boots, and a shotgun, blasting people. She has a written hit list of most-hated politician's and other public figures of the day (Robert Mugabe, the Burmese generals, and so on). One by one she would have the phantom with the gun shoot them down, while lying on her back being zapped.

"It was so good; it was quite cathartic," she confided. The staff were astonished to find her often grinning after the treatment, where most people were reeling!

[It might seem crude and violent for such a nice lady; but to me, I see the merit in this. We all have bottled up rage and anger which, for obvious social reasons must be kept in check. But to imagine ourselves free to do violence and hit back at things gives us a surge of power and release. I'm OK with it, really.]

"When I'm feeling down, I get the list out and have a good laugh," she giggled to Vivien and me. "So much bloodshed, so few tears!" She showed us the list. From the relish with which she spoke about this technique—and in fact she said as much herself—this was probably Tash's single most effective creative visualization and helped her conquest of the disease the most. "Get in touch with your inner sadist," she joked!

Knowing what I know of the destructive powers of buried anger and resentment, I'm sure she's right.

The lady was so funny and perceptive. I could have listened to her shrewd observations for hours. Before we left, Tash shared some of her poetry and cartoons. No question, hers was a scintillating, dynamic and creative intellect. If her accent made me think of Scottish dourness, her lively, jokey, almost flippant wit soon got me past that. She made Viv and I laugh generously.

[I think Tash laughs at fate and may she have many more years of life. I am planning to try and persuade her to a trans-Atlantic recorded interview for my followers.... but she describes herself as a hopeless Luddite, where technology is concerned]

Oppose Family Pressures

Close family are not always supportive and helpful. Many of them stupidly believe all the propaganda about cancer treatments and the claims that we are "winning the war." Statistics say otherwise.

In any case, the issue is not one of being compelled to adopt the "best" line of treatment. It's actually about your right to choose. With very few exceptions, the law allows you the right to follow a path that you set. Remember, most physicians are not allowed the right to choose how to treat you; they could end up in jail for not sticking to the party line. But you—the patient—can still agree or not agree with what is proposed by an oncologist.

If Sis starts screaming and weeping and wringing her hands, demanding that you MUST follow the path (of orthodox medicine) realize she is dramatizing her own fears rather than concerns for you. She has a guilt package running or extreme anxiety that she will get drawn into what *could have* happened, if you don't toe the line. Harsh—but true, I'm afraid.

Learn To Say No!

One of the important aspects of "recovering" from being a meek and mild cancer personality type is that you have GOT to stop being a doormat for people. You must learn to say "No!" If people don't get it, dump them. If you can't dump them because you are married to him/her, or it's some other family member, explain curtly but sweetly that you now need time to take care of yourself. If he or she still doesn't get it, try shouting it at the top of your voice!

Why am I emphasizing this and asking you to do something that is almost certain to cause tension, if not trouble and conflict? Because it's for your survival.

One significant study showed that people who learned to say "No" and stop being a people-pleaser lived significantly longer than people who made no changes. That tells you two things:

1. Saying "Yes" to things you don't like is a bad idea and can actually be lethal.

2. Making significant mental and attitude changes can enhance your survival, no matter what disease you are facing down.

That's not to say that I want you to become obnoxious to those around you. Simply that you start drawing some lines and then *enforce them*. People who love you should fall into line very quickly; they just need a few pointers and an occasional reminder. Those who don't respect your boundaries, no matter your urgings, are actually toxic people and you should eliminate them from your surroundings.

Is this your spouse? No matter; you need to get rid of such individuals, to ensure your survival. "Getting rid" of a spouse can be a case of taking a break, having a vacation alone, visiting with other members of the family or making a point of being out of the home evenings, when he or she is usually home.

Just get cunning, OK? It's very important.

Push Back Against Bullying

Opposition may not come from just family and friends. Many oncologists are abusive rogues and even threaten their patients; some even get angry and rage at the person supposedly in their care (oh yes, it happens!) Often he or she will resort to the dirty trick of lying and claiming you will die if you don't do what they say. That is evil.

Demand they show the survival figures if you did comply. Often a miserable round of chemo will statistically provide little more than a few extra months. For the patient it is Hell. The only happy person is the oncologist, who gets the money!

But remember, you are not a statistic. You are a determined, motivated individual and facts show that such people survive far better than the average patient.

Oncologist Bernie Siegel, in his lovely book *Love, Medicine and Miracles*, tells us that patients who are cussed or ornery (indomitable and intransigent, if you want some clever words) do far better that those who are polite and wouldn't dream of telling a doctor to f**k off.

A research team with the CRC Psychological Medicine Group, Royal Marsden Hospital, Surrey, UK under Steven Greer, also found that cancer patients who had a "fighting spirit" lived longer. In this study high levels of anger correlated with better outcome, and patients who felt helpless or hopeless did poorly. These studies are showing us that a patient's will to live or fighting spirit has a great deal to do with chances for recovery. . [Greer S, Morris T,

Pettingale KW, Haybittle JL. Psychological response to breast cancer and 15-year outcome. Lancet. 1990 Jan 6;335(8680):49–50.]

Surprisingly, those who engaged in denial had a better chance of survival than those who felt hopeless. Denial included saying such things as, "I didn't have cancer. The doctor only removed my breast as a precautionary measure."

A ten-year follow-up confirmed the original findings. Of those who showed a fighting spirit or denied they had cancer, 55 percent were still alive, compared with 22 percent of those who had a helpless/hopeless response or engaged in stoic acceptance. But why would denial help? Apparently patients who deny they have cancer feel better and adjust better than those who give up and feel utterly hopeless.

Well, denial is really only a version of affirmations, isn't it, where we state something that is not true as if it were completely true? "I am rich beyond my wildest dreams, I own a red Ferrari Testarossa, etc. is only like saying "Cancer has no power over me. No tumor can survive in my body but will be swept away with natural healing processes..." What's the difference?

Consider this inspiring account of survival from one of the worst of all cancers:

WILLFUL OBLIVION

At Brain Blogger, Lisa Reisman tells us how she was officially cured of brain cancer—specifically, a glioblastoma multiforme (GBM), the most lethal of brain tumors.

According to the *Journal of Neuroepidemiology*, a "population-based cure is thought to occur when a population's risk of death returns to that of the normal population, and in GBM, that is thought to occur after 10 years."

Wisely, she didn't put much stock in statistics, neither when she got her diagnosis sixteen years ago nor since. She practiced a version of the art of denial she called "willful oblivion."

Lisa shares with us her coping strategies and I, for one, find them instructional and well worth sharing. With the caveat that there is no-one-size-fits-all approach to contending with the diagnosis of a serious illness, here are three.

1. Lies, Damned Lies, and Statistics

Glioblastoma multiforme is certainly not a good call, with a median survival rate of one to two years.

Lisa didn't know the statistics and didn't need to. She asked not to be told her prognosis. There was a feeling that being told such facts when you are in a state of extreme dread, that anything said to you will be seared into the mind and become "true" for that reason (if only oncologists recognized this and stopped giving stupid prognostications, "You have three months to live, maybe six..." becomes a self-fulfilling prophecy, not a statistical truth.

"One to two years to live," she tells us, "Would have been seared into my mind. The clock would have started ticking."

Evolutionary biologist Stephen Jay Gould had a far more refined reproach. In July 1982, as he recounts in his 1985 essay "The Median Isn't the Message," he learned he was suffering from abdominal mesothelioma, a rare and toxic cancer usually associated with exposure to asbestos, with a median survival of eight months after discovery.

The news was devastating. But then Gould began doing some digging. As someone trained in statistics, he distinguished *median survival*, a measure commonly used to express survival rates, as the amount of time after which 50% of the patients have died and 50% have survived.

In other words, a median survival rate of eight months didn't mean he had eight months to live. Given his relative youth — he was forty — the superlative medical treatment he knew he would receive, and his generally "sanguine" attitude, it meant there was no reason he could not be among the latter 50%. Above all, he recognized the near impossibility at diagnosis of knowing whether any individual will place to the left of the median — that is to say, before the eight months for his particular illness — or the right, after the eight months.

This was where he found solace. With his particular makeup, he could imagine himself surviving far out along the right of the median. And that's precisely what he did. Following surgery and experimental chemotherapy, he lived twenty more years before dying, in 2002, at the age of sixty, from a lung cancer unrelated to his original disease.

Doctors and Big Pharma are fond of manipulating figures in their favor. Well, here's proof that manipulating them in YOUR favor can work wonders!

2.   **The Unsung Benefits of Denial**

Walk into any oncology ward; you will see the gray skin, the eyes the color of dull pennies, the puffy features. That's the face of cancer. Lisa Reisman looked away and would have none of it. During chemotherapy treatments, she insisted on being treated in a small alcove separated from the main ward.

Her mission was simple: to view herself not as an inhabitant in the world of cancer but as someone who happened to be in treatment for cancer but would continue, to the extent possible, to go about the routines of daily living in the land of the well.

It's important to note that this wasn't the form of denial that Anna Freud described as an unconscious defense against painful and overwhelming aspects of external reality. That denial has been generally viewed as a pathological, ineffective defense mechanism. It could get you killed.

Even an article on the Mayo Clinic website, while acknowledging that "short-term denial … gives your mind the opportunity to unconsciously absorb shocking or distressing information at a pace that won't send you into a psychological tailspin," warns that "denial should only be a temporary measure — it won't change the reality of the situation" and counsels those stuck in the denial phase to consider talking to a mental health provider.

Of course, the kind of denial to which the Mayo Clinic refers is a folly that one *does not have* a disease, leading the patient to refuse any treatment, holistic or otherwise. But recent studies propose shifting the lens on the concept of denial—specifically, as an adaptive strategy in meeting the impact of the disease.

A review in the Journal of Psycho-Oncology exploring denial in cancer patients found that "denial was related to improved psychological functioning." Those patients deployed "active strategies of realizing that one s cancer, but choosing not to let the illness control their lives, trying to ush the illness aside, and instead create a positive outlook."

Ruth McCorkle, a pioneer in oncology nursing and professor of epidemiology at Yale, had this take: "Some patients compartmentalize their disease," she recently told me. "It's a way to shield themselves from paralyzing fear and at the same time remain functional."

3. **Practicing Denial As An Adaptive Strategy**

In view of his positive outcome, let's return to Gould's essay — specifically, the reply from Sir Peter Medawar, his personal scientific guru and a Nobel laureate in immunology, when he questioned him on the best prescription for success against cancer. "A sanguine personality," Sir Peter replied (sanguine: calm, not easily ruffled, adaptive, optimistic or positive, especially in an apparently bad or difficult situation).

That was in keeping with Gould's thinking. "In general," he wrote, "those with positive attitudes, with a strong will and purpose for living, with commitment to struggle, with an active response to aiding their own treatment and not just a passive acceptance of anything doctors say, tend to live longer."

Ruth McCorkle went further. "It's about continuing to go about your routine. It's choosing not to say I can no longer do this because I have cancer or even why should I continue to do this as someone with cancer and instead saying 'why not try to do what I can?' It's about asserting control over circumstances."

Lisa Reisman added extra daily tasks, to take her mind off the negative possibilities. She adopted a maxim from her high school cross-country coach. When facing a seemingly insurmountable challenge, break it down into manageable distances, he'd say.

In other words, set achievable goals each day. Walking, for example. Walk 500 steps or, if you're feeling a bit worn down, 100 steps, or even 50. Memorize a poem. If you're not up to a whole poem, memorize one line. Or two. Draw a picture, or an outline of a picture. Work on a crossword puzzle. Try solving one clue. If you're not up to more, put it aside.

There's a fluidity to this regimen. The one essential: make a commitment to do what you choose as your activities every day, even if it's just a pale approximation of what you might do if you were entirely well.

Why? Because, as McCorkle suggested, it's a way of compartmentalizing your disease. It's a way of creating your own sustainable reality within your self that the truth is what you make it. You generate your world, not mindless statistics.

Resilience does not mean that one is forced into thinking positively all of the time. For many years, having a positive attitude was strongly emphasized because it was believed that attitudes might affect survival. This assumption is not without controversy, but most studies show that feigning a relentlessly positive attitude may actually become an added stressor.

Studies suggest it may be perfectly OK to be sad and angry, and not unusual to find patients (even for those who cope well) bargaining for survival with a higher Being. It's also normal to have great days in which people feel positive toward life, to pace themselves with what they can do when they are feeling well and commit to achievable goals.

References:

[http://brainblogger.com/2015/05/04/denial-an-unorthodox-strategy-for-coping-with-cancer-diagnosis/]

Courneya KS, Mackey JR, & Jones LW (2000). Coping with cancer: can exercise help? The Physician and sportsmedicine, 28 (5), 49-73 PMID: 20086640

Gould, Stephen Jay (1985). The Median Isn't the Message. Accessed online 29 April 2015.

Smoll NR, Schaller K, & Gautschi OP (2012). The cure fraction of glioblastoma multiforme. Neuroepidemiology, 39 (1), 63-9 PMID: 22776797

Is All This Worth The Effort?

Maybe you are not convinced and are still wondering if it is really worth the effort? After all, there are lots of claims that it's all a waste of time; that there is nothing you can do about cancer; that psychology and attitude are proven to be irrelevant or unworkable (not true but a common claim).

Alastair J Cunningham, Professor Emeritus at Toronto University and author of *The Healing Journey* set out to investigate how taking charge of your life can help, not just with cancer but any disease. The book is a practical guide for people who wish to address a diagnosis of cancer not just as a biological disease, but also as a psychological and spiritual crisis. Cunningham took 22 patients with various kinds of supposedly incurable cancer. After asking experts to predict each patient's life-span, he and his team painstakingly gathered data on each participant's attitudes and behaviors as they participated in an intervention along the lines of the earlier experiment.

The result? Cunningham found that patients who worked the hardest at transforming themselves psychologically—lived *at least three times longer than predicted*. That's awesome. Triple the predicted survival rate?

The sad side of the story is that, with one or two exceptions, the least active died right on schedule. "It makes sense to me that the people who live longer are those who make substantial psychological changes," says Cunningham. "Of course, only a few do that."

Cunningham's discovery won't stop the debate about psychological interventions' impact on patients' life spans. Scientists still don't even know how cancer develops. "For years we've been puzzling around the labs trying to figure out what regulates cancer," says Cunningham, noting that the endocrine or immune systems may play a role. "Not much is known yet."

General: Br J Cancer. 1998 Jun; 77(12): 2381–2385

There's plenty more of that sort:

A study of attitudes in patients with malignant melanoma showed that stoic acceptance in women and helplessness/hopelessness in men were associated with poorer outcome. Emotional expression, even expression of so-called negative emotions, may be good for one's health by buffering the possible negative effects of distress and depression.

A study that carefully reviewed the evidence related to emotional and psychosocial factors affecting cancer patients concluded that the "inability to express emotion, particularly in relation to anger" is a real factor contributing to the progress of a cancer. Those patients who repressed their emotions had a greater likelihood that their cancer would grow and spread.

In fact researchers have found that one of the body's "happy" neurotransmitters forces some cancer cells to commit suicide. They say that when serotonin is placed in a test tube alongside tumor cells of Burkitt's lymphoma the cancer undergoes apoptosis (programmed cell death): "An exciting property of serotonin is that it can tell some cells to self-destruct. We have found serotonin can get inside the lymphoma cells and instruct them to commit suicide."

It is already known that Prozac and other SSRIs reduce the incidence of colon cancer. I'm not a supporter of SSRIs but let's think of them as "happy pills". Isn't is confirming the psycho-neurological hypothesis of cancer, that these happy pills lessen the risk of cancer? [World J Gastrointest Oncol. 2014 Jan 15; 6(1): 11−21. Published online 2014 Jan 15.

However, it's not all good. Prozac is unlikely to ever establish itself as a cancer treatment! Take note...

An international team of researchers led by John Gordon, professor of immunology at Birmingham University, found evidence to suggest cancer cells can be killed by "positive thinking", but which is then *blocked* by taking Prozac. That's bad. But it still emphasizes the psycho-neurological connection, doesn't it? I think so.

The Birmingham study examined the effects of Prozac and other antidepressants on a group of tumor cells growing in a test tube. The researchers found that the drug prevented the cancer cells from committing "suicide", thereby leading to a more vigorous growth of the tumors. This is assumed to be because Prozac blocks serotonin pathways.

Although an increased risk of cancer has not so far been detected in Prozac patients, the latest findings could lead to a global re-evaluation of the drug's long-term safety.

The research work was designed to find new ways of treating lymphomas, a type of blood cancer, by investigating how the brain communicates with the immune system to induce "positive thinking" through the neuro-transmitter serotonin.

Serotonin is a natural chemical that regulates people's moods, keeping them balanced. Too much serotonin affects appetite and sleep and too little affects the mood, perhaps causing depression. It is a surprise to many (including me) that serotonin can get inside the lymphoma cells and instruct them to commit suicide, thereby providing the potential for an effective therapy.

If this is true, then we have a plausible scientific mechanism as to how positive thinking can slow or stem cancer growth. Feeling good means serotonin; serotonin gets inside cancer cells; serotonin causes the cells to self-destruct.

It would also make sense that Prozac and other SSRIs such as Paxil and Celexa had the effect of stimulating the growth of at least one tumor, known as Burkitt's lymphoma. [Blood, April 1, 2002, Vol. 99, No. 7, pp. 2545-2553]

Watch this space!

POSITIVE PSYCHOLOGY

Historically, psychology and psychiatry have been about studying the weird and abnormal.

There's been a definite thrust in recent years towards studying the psychology of feeling good and getting positive outcomes in life, rather than problems. My own Supernoetics® has the Protocols For Change and Human Transformation™ that play very positively into this area.

But the acknowledged "guru" of positive psychology, as it's called, is Dr. Martin Seligman. In *Authentic Happiness: Using the New Positive Psychology to Realize Your Potential for Lasting Fulfillment* he makes the point: "Relieving the states that make life miserable... has made building the states that make life worth living less of a priority."

The time has finally arrived for a science that seeks to understand positive emotion, build strength and virtue, and provide guideposts for finding what Aristotle called the 'good life'".

Seligman advises us to achieve emotional fulfillment and increase one's "happiness quotient" through pursuing one's innate strengths and incorporating strengths such as humor, originality and generosity into everyday interactions, rather than picking apart the past, trying to solve decades-old problems and to fix weaknesses.

Positive feelings, as we have been seeing, may be a key to effective cancer cures.

Here are 5 suggestions for working towards a positive psychology in your life:

Below are a few exercises that can be used in practice to help clients live a more thriving and flourishing life.

Look For Your Strengths

We all have attributes, skills, and talents that can be developed further, and focusing on these areas can provide us continued confidence and purpose. Write down at least five talents or strengths that you are aware of in yourself.

Write down five further talents or strengths you would like to develop. Pick *just one* and get started on that, whether it's painting, dance, building models, reading Jane Austen, or whatever.

You can also answer the Via Institute on Character questionnaire online at this web address: http://www.viacharacter.org/www

Look For Optimism

Just as hopeful and helpless thinking patterns are learned over time, so too can people learn to think more optimistically. Try to become aware of your thinking patterns and to recognize the type of statements that provide a positive and optimistic outlook. Eliminate the negative.

Self-Direction And Purpose

We all dream of being at our best and achieving our potential, so exploring your dreams and aspirations can get you thinking of the kind of life you truly desire.

There is a version of this from "Solutions Focus" (looking from the solution angle, instead of looking at the problem), called the miracle question: "What would be different in your life if you woke up and by some miracle everything you ever wanted, everything good you could ever imagine for yourself, had actually happened?"

What would you see? How would you know everything had come true? It's a great exercize and very inspiring.

A Gratitude Journal or Logbook

Gratitude is a magnificent mood enhancer. Instead of thinking what you don't have, rejoice in what you DO have! The things we are grateful for can be easily overlooked, unless we consciously focus on them. Deciding what we are grateful for and writing it down can be an effective means to increase our self-esteem and our view of life. This can be done by designating a few days a week to write down four or five things we are grateful for, whether from that day or in general.

As you grow into this, you could try writing a letter to someone who you are very grateful to but have never expressed your appreciation of them. This gets stronger if you read the letter out loud, pretending you are speaking to that person.

Mindfulness And Savoring Positivity

One of the commonly shared beneficial changes when you are faced with your mortality is that every moment becomes more precious. Cancer cases will often enthusiastically describe how they are slowing down and staying present and how that helps increase positive emotions. This could be at times like eating a meal, showering, or going for a walk. Really experience the moment and fully engage in your day to day undertakings.

I also highly recommend you read *Happier* by Tal Ben-Shahar (McGraw-Hill, New York, 2007)

No matter how much time you have left on Earth, you cannot do better than focus on what is important to you. As the great psychologist Carl Jung wrote: "The least of things with a meaning is worth more in life than the greatest of things without it."

Here's a simple hack from Ben-Shahar's book to help focus you further:

Draw a circle. Label that "Can do."

Draw a smaller circle inside that and label it: "Want to do."

Draw an even smaller circle inside that and label it: "Really want to do."

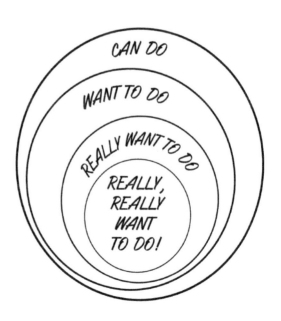

Finally draw an inner circle you will label: "Really, *really* want to do."

It isn't even necessary to fill in the outer three circles; you get the point! Focus all your life, earnestly, in what you put in that innermost circle. It's the whole meaning of your life. Let it be your passion!

JOURNALING

Obviously, navigating your way through a cancer journey can be tough. It can be hard to find time to care for your body, spirit and mind.

Storytelling is one of our most fundamental and enduring needs. Our stories define us. They are the vehicles of meaning and they serve as the narrative of our views about our world and ourselves. We all constantly tell stories that shape virtually every human activity from our emotions to our personal relationships and our politics. One of the casualties of the pharmacological eclipse of the "talk therapies," has been that many people are no longer being encouraged to explore the meaning of their distress.

Journaling is one way to tell your story and reflect on your journey. It's surprisingly cathartic (catharsis is the releasing of pent up emotions). Writing down your thoughts gives you an opportunity to work out your feelings and emotions, which may help you relax and find reasons to be happier and more hopeful about the future.

A surprising amount of research has been done on the effects of journaling, most notably by James W. Pennebaker, Liberal Arts Professor of Psychology at the University of Texas at Austin. He began investigations in the late 1980s with the study of the effect of writing on rape victims, and his research convincingly suggests expressive writing about emotional upheavals in our lives can improve our physical and mental health.

Many other researchers have investigated this subject and have made equally profound discoveries. Simply put, journaling enhances healing: mental *and physical* healing, take note. Just knowing this can offer additional hope and motivation to reluctant writers.

It's a very strong tool that most cancer patients would benefit from learning to use.

Methods Of Journaling

The MD Anderson Cancer Center website (www.mdanderson.org) gives several types of journaling you might want to explore:

Gratitude journaling: Write down everything you're grateful for. This focuses your attention on positive aspects of your life.

Blog: A blog is a website that you can easily update by writing short posts. Blog posts can be as simple as commentary on your day-to-day life and treatment, or reflection pieces exploring your life's purpose or connecting with a higher power.

Stream-of-consciousness writing: Write down everything that comes to your mind. This unstructured, unedited writing will reflect your raw thoughts and observations.

Art journaling: Draw, doodle or scrapbook what you're feeling and thinking.

Line-a-day journaling: Limit yourself to a single line or sentence for the day.

The Benefits Of Journaling

There's no right or wrong way to journal. Research shows that taking as little as 20 minutes a month for 3 months, to write, will produce long lasting benefits to your physical and emotional health.

Journaling can help you sleep better, reduce fatigue and help you adjust psychologically to a cancer diagnosis and treatment.

Look for the positive: Journaling can help you identify positive situations or events that have unfolded due to your cancer diagnosis. You may have been reunited with a loved one, received an outpouring of support from friends, co-workers and family, or been able to warn others about dangerous lifestyle habits. Documenting these areas in writing may help you explore and appreciate them more.

Look for what you can control: Journaling can also help you map out and decide what things you can and do have control over and how you can use that knowledge in your life.

Find peace in your relationships: Journaling privately can even help with your day-to-day social interactions. Disclosing your deepest feelings in writing might prepare you to have a difficult conversation with a loved one, or it might allow you to simply enjoy your time together without worrying about nagging negative thoughts.

Tips For Journaling

Journal for yourself. There is no wrong way to do it as long as it is beneficial to you.

Find a quiet space. Make sure you journal during a time you know you won't be interrupted for at least 20 minutes. Find a safe, secure and comfortable area to work.

Don't worry about grammar, spelling or sentence structure. No one will read this without your consent, so it doesn't have to be perfect. Focus on the subject of your writing: What are you feeling? What thoughts come to mind as you recall these events? What do you want to make sure you don't forget?

And another important piece of advice: Protect your thoughts and writings. If writing by hand, keep your journal in a safe spot where someone won't spill something on it or read your thoughts without your consent. If you are typing your journal, password protect the document to keep it away from prying eyes.

Seek professional help. If journaling about experiences and emotions leaves you more upset than relieved, meet with a social worker or mental health professional and use your journal to introduce what's bothering you.

You can also seek aid through my unexploded ® piloting program, which is specifically geared to lifting the heavy stress elements in a person's psychological make up. Let's look at that next...

HEAVY LIFTING PSYCHOLOGY

Remember you read in the section about Dr. Hamer's work (page 22) that cancer often follows a shocking psychic trauma. Bad things lead to bad things, like a wound leading to a scar.

We are, in a certain sense, defined by our most traumatic experiences. We can, at times, soar to the heights and feel great; a truly joyful dimension of Being. But these wonderful enhanced spiritual moments don't seem to last. They are very wonderful but ephemeral and impact our lives very little, compared to the effect of dark, negative experiences.

That's not meant to say we are not enriched by the good times. But we are much more defined by our lowest moments.

That's a problem.

But there is good in this too. It means we can inch ourselves upwards, degree by degree, by taking and eradicating the blackness of the bad times. It can be done. In fact there have been numerous methods over the years. I merely submit to you that the latest incarnation of such techniques—my Supernoetics® "piloting"—is far advanced as a technique.

I'm now going to step over certain therapies which are popular but are clearly not working at a deep enough level; methods like EMDR (eye movement desensitization and reprocessing), EFT (emotional freedom technique) and Lester Levenson's Releasing Technique®, later reworked by Hale Dwoskin as The Sedona Method.

That's not to say these approaches have no value. But I can't count the number of people I have encountered who claim to have used one of these techniques and yet are still sad and clearly in pain when their key topic is addressed.

What is clear to me and my colleagues is that these cheery, simple approaches merely persuade a person to take their minds away from the pain. It's like dealing with an unexploded bomb by walling it off. There's still an unexploded bomb behind the barrier. It's not truly "dealt with" till the fuse is taken out and the bomb is no longer able to explode.

So it is, that many a time I have had a case say, "I dealt with the issue of my father's abuse," and yet within minutes she was bawling freely when asked the details. In other words, it was not dealt with and had never gone away. She had just successfully walled it off; put it behind a wall of justifications, politically-correct explanations, and wrong thinking.

Without getting too technical in so short a text, the issue is one of truth, or what, in Supernoetics®, we call the Deep-ISness (an other-worldly realm of knowing that is far below the surface). The *real* truth, if you like.

When that is contacted things change… a lot. We call it shift. It means seeing life anew, from a completely fresh perspective.

So, for example, the abuse case often plays out something like the following:

A woman has been seeing a "therapist" for years, dealing with childhood abuse. She has talked and talked and talked about it. All the time it gets more solid, instead of slowly evaporating. Having been fed garbage notions from the therapist, she now has all sorts of reasons why her life is screwed up. The unexploded bomb is now coated with layer upon layer of chocolate, marzipan, toffee and marshmallows!

She comes to see me and, after sending her back in time with a propri-etary technique called Hypnoetics™ (yes, not too different from hypnotism) she discharges some grief. With a little gentle probing—or guidance-style technique that we call "piloting", meaning navigating—we find surprising thoughts stuck to the original memories.

She is still "back then", which is critical to catharsis. With very little help she finds a thought she had never dared think before: *mother did not help me*. Mother should have intervened and saved her. Mother did not. There-fore mother betrayed her. Now she's seeing this from the inner child's point of view, remember. Usually by now (I've had many of these cases), she is shocked to find herself angry with mother.

But she now has a new dimension to her woes, previously unsuspected; one that is healing and releases her pent up misery.

She has undergone a major shift. Suddenly the scenario is not horrible father but uncaring, enabling mother who didn't put a stop to it (co-dependence, so-called). Once in a while mother even emerges as a provocateur, driving father to violent acts. Those mothers have a lot to answer for.

Well, of course it plays out eventually. The patient realizes that the healing that never took place was to forgive her mother for failing her in a time need. Yapping on about father, as therapists are wont to do, achieved nothing. It missed an important deeper truth, the Deep-IS. Big bullying father did not heal anything, it just recycled the pain; silly, incompetent mother did heal it, all gone!

Sometimes, indeed, there are gales of laughter, as the patient realizes how much she has been suppressing herself by holding these painful memories of years gone by right in front of her own face! It is rather like using the traumatic past as a pair of goggles, through which to view the world. It distorts everything.

So you can multiply this approach a thousand-fold and imagine cases of accidents, trauma, near-death experiences, diseases, murder, loss, wartime experiences, and the whole panoply of human ills. We seem to hypnotize ourselves with painful, buried memories. Only the truth (the Deep-IS truth) can set a person free.

The rule I have evolved is this: if the person has a psychological problem, with a satisfactory "explanation" of how it arose, that is entirely incorrect! *The true origin of a problem will see it vanish in a trice. Poof!* No more psychological problem or pain—like in the illustrative case I just gave you, where relations with mother and father are fully healed.

Sometimes it is just a matter of skill, finding something that everyone else had missed. I remember a case of a woman with a malignant brain tumor. Her memory of childhood was a complete blank, up to the age of around seven years. She was outstandingly cold and unemotional. Her loving husband often found it difficult to break through this and get to intimate physical acts.

With the Hypnoetics™ approach, she uncovered dreadful memories that had remained deeply buried. As a child of about four years old, she began to recall being led by her grandfather to a cabin in the woods. There she was stripped, tied down, and raped repeatedly by a group of men (including the grandfather).

Afterwards she was sworn to secrecy and told to forget all about it; if she ever told a soul what had happened in the cabin in the woods, they would murder her.

So, she dutifully blanked out her childhood memories. She could remember nothing at all before the age of seven years. Of course, the whole ghastly event was still imprinted deep in her psyche; the fuse was not removed from the unexploded bomb.

So eventually, it went off! Bang! She got a brain tumor.

The remainder of this story is a happy one. Her tumor markers rapidly regressed. Eventually all signs of the growth disappeared on the MRI scan. She made a remarkable recovery. Incidentally, she also warmed in her emotions and became far more feminine and responsive to the advances of her delighted husband!

This lady, now in her forties, was outstandingly confident that she had un-covered the real "cause" of her cancer. I shuddered to hear that she would not change her diet or even take nutritional supplements! The bomb was totally defused, as far as she was concerned. But I'm still nervous around explosives...

If you want to explore what Supernoetics® piloting can do to heal your life, get in touch. Start by emailing Vivien at scottmumbywellness@gmail.com

OK, moving on...

FIND A SUPPORT TEAM

You don't have to go through cancer alone. If people around you are relent-lessly negative and trying to tell you to knuckle under and do as you are told, you may need to retreat into your own space (you have read that acquiescent patients do not fare as well as the feisty ones).

But a better idea is to put together a positive support team; a group of peo-ple who will share the worries and the burdens; maybe even run errands for you; reminds you about schedules and perhaps even take over some of your chores. Also a team can keep you on track, cheer you up on gloomy days and listen to your deep inner thoughts as these surface throughout the crisis.

Actually two support teams! The first would be a support and comfort team, and the other a psycho-medical team. A support and comfort team may be family and close friends, a social worker and even clergy. A psycho-medical team might consist of oncologists, surgeons, nurse practitioners, bedside nurses and a licensed psychologist or a psychiatrist.

I have already remarked that even holistic regimens can be tough. The Ger-son Therapy is nothing less than heroic—juicing day and night, tons of sup-plements to swallow, coffee enemas several times a day... it isn't for people who lack self discipline, or who don't like carrots, and you have to be pretty firm with yourself to keep to the hyper strict vegan, plant-based, no salt and virtually fat-free diet.

Group Therapy

Similar to a support team is signing up for group therapy. The main difference is that group therapy sessions are led and (usually) someone has to pay, somewhere.

Psychiatrist David Spiegel, M.D., of the Stanford University School of Medicine, launched the debate about whether psycho-social interventions can lengthen lives in 1989, when he published a now-classic paper describing his work with breast cancer patients.

In the study, patients came together in weekly group therapy sessions to express their feelings about cancer and receive support from fellow victims. When Spiegel followed up a decade later, he discovered that patients who had participated in the sessions had survived an average of 18 months longer than those in the control group.

Years of controversy have followed, with researchers trying—with mixed results—to replicate Spiegel's findings.

It seems a no-brainer to me, since you don't need scientific "proof" that group togetherness can be supportive.

However—and this is the real kicker—*you need a good, caring, supportive group leader and the members need to be positive too.* You might think it strange I am saying this. But far too often I have seen patients broken and hurt after attending group therapy with an arrogant, judgmental know-all in charge (or a dominant group member who takes on this attitude). Such a person is very destructive and apparently seeks to run her (or his) management and validation issues on others, sneering at those who won't (or those who will) adopt orthodox treatments.

The wrong sort of group therapy environment, with faulty control factors is, in my opinion, the probable reason that some studies have sometimes failed to show any benefits from group therapy.

One paper, published in 1973, thoroughly examined the impact of leadership style on intensive small group casualties. The charismatic leaders who were overly confronting, pressuring members for immediate and highly personal self-disclosure, and who imposed their values on the participants, often failed to recognize crumbling defenses in fragile members.

The researchers found that attack or other rejection of a member by the group (or leader) was among the primary mechanisms of injury.

[Lieberman M, Yalom I, Miles M: Encounter Groups: First Facts. New York, Basic Books, 1973]

So be warned. Go along to a weekly meeting if it suits. But be sure to sit on the sidelines for a couple of visits, and refuse to be drawn in, until you sense its style and leadership. Of course if the leader or any member mocks you for being hesitant, that's a clear signal you are not going to get any benefit and may find yourself wounded in the process.

A "Psychic Support Group"

This might sound a strange idea. What I am referring to is the possibility of finding helpers at the psychological or imaginative level. Many people feel the strong presence of a psychic being, who is aware of their issues and seems to be able to offer guidance. Even oncologist Bernie Siegel (see page 15) admits he has "spirit guides" or helpers, as they are sometime called.

Siegel met his personal guide, George, attending a workshop with Carl and Stephanie Simonton, when he was told during a guided imagery exercise he would meet an inner guide. The orthodox mechanic-style doctor in Siegel said, "This is all ridiculous."

And yet, in the meditation, along came George. George is a spiritual figure occupying inner space, who now guides Bernie. Since then Siegel has met other "guides". He admits he can only see the guides in imagery exercises, and sense them nearby, but he has been assured by mediums they can really see these guides, standing around him while giving lectures or workshops.

A new world opened up where a mechanic could exist no longer with the old belief systems. The new outlook turned Siegel into one of the most humanitarian and wise oncologists on the planet. He has been named one of the top 20 Spiritually Influential Living People on the Planet by the Watkins Review which is published by Watkins Books, an esoteric bookshop in the heart of London, England.

So don't knock "spirit guides"!

Cancer survivor Marc Ian Barasch, author of The Healing Path describing his own journey to conquer cancer, writes of a "mythic helper."

"The helper often seems to spark a startling cognitive shift in the way the journeyer relates to disease, as well as to shake up the existing patterns of life. He or she may push the patient toward "shadow-work", helping to uncover rejected parts of the self that, long sequestered in darkness, contain powers of both sickness and healing." Marc Ian Barasch, *The Healing Path*, p. 245.

You may have an intuition about yours. But you can always search, using guided imagery, until you find your guide who—I believe—will naturally be waiting there for you to show up and probably ask you, "What took you so long?"

Others will consider anything but the help of Jesus as being worthless. It's all just perspective.

THERAPEUTIC LAUGHTER

Most of us are familiar with the extraordinary book *The Anatomy Of An Illness* by Normal Cousins (1979). In it he describes the therapeutic benefits of laughter. Cousins had crippling arthritis and was told, pretty much, it was incurable.

Well, it wasn't! He checked out a whole bunch of old movies (Marx Brothers, Candid Camera Episodes, The Three Stooges, Laurel and Hardy, etc.) and laughed his head off for weeks and months.

The result? His arthritis was cured. He later wrote about his success with this approach and recovery for the *New England Journal of Medicine*. Doctors studiously ignored his "unscientific" suggestion, of course. They put their faith—to this day—in "treatments" that cure nothing and are in themselves dangerous (opioid deaths have now reached epidemic proportions).

Extending Cousins Idea

Here's something that goes beyond *The Anatomy Of An Illness* and has therapeutic potential for all of us. The things is, Cousins set himself up with a good reason to laugh: comedy movies.

But what if there is no "reason" to laugh? Well, there is always a reason to laugh, if you look around you! It can be, in itself, a mental weakness to always need a reason to do things. Spontaneity (no reason) is, in itself, an end or reason and can be highly therapeutic for us all!

Try this:

Just stand up and start laughing—WITHOUT ANY REASON AT ALL!

At first you may find it incredibly difficult. We all feel we need a reason to laugh (or do anything else). You don't.

To do anything without a reason can be soothing and enhancing. It is an ability we need to develop. Otherwise life becomes much too serious.

When you get going and find you can start laughing at will and without a cause, next push yourself to keep laughing! And don't get serious about it. Don't try too hard. Forget about laughing authentically. Just laugh!

You will find other changes will take place in your mental landscape, other than just a more joyous sense of humor. You won't be as stressed or anxious about outcomes; you'll be able to open up to other points of view; what once seemed a problem will recede; people you couldn't stand will become tolerable.

Here's a tip: you'll find it incredibly easier to do this if you stand in front of a mirror. The bathroom is a good place to start your laughter workshop. If you can't hack it with laughter at first, just smile! It feels wonderful to have that you-in-the-mirror smiling warmly back at you.

Within a day or two you'll find yourself able to laugh!

One of my friends who I shared this with remembered an experience from her youth:

> Dear Dr. Keith, what a fun idea, thank you! It reminds me of when I was young and my friends and I had a little game of going to a party or a restaurant and starting to 'group laugh'. If all went to plan, within a short time, nearly everyone around us was either laughing or smiling. On one occasion a waiter came over to our table and said that a gentleman wanted to know what we were laughing about. We said 'absolutely nothing' and when the waiter relayed the message the gentleman smiled and gestured us his approval and offered to buy us all a drink! That was our biggest success.

It's been said before and said often: laughter is infectious. It's also very therapeutic!

It cleans up unpleasant relationships. You can add this to your mirror routine: mock up the presence of people you hate or have difficulty with. Laugh at them! Laugh long and loud at these people and bring them down to a confrontable presence. If you are a woman who has been slighted and abused by men, laugh at them in the mirror and tell them what fools they were to miss out on a honey like you! (need I say that men can do this too?)

Science? Oh yes!

Whether we giggle, chortle, chuckle, guffaw or "lol" (laughing out loud), everyone laughs. Smiling, a natural part of laughing, is a universal indication of happiness or pleasure across all cultures.

When we smile, the brain releases dopamine, a neurotransmitter that produces feelings of happiness. Interestingly enough, this effect works both ways: the release of dopamine when we feel happy causes us to smile, and the mere act of smiling causes the brain to release dopamine, which in turn makes us feel happy.

The results of many scientific studies on the effects of laughter have led most experts to agree that laughter can be remarkably therapeutic. For example, laughter and humor have been shown to increase tolerance to pain. Additionally, researchers in Japan have found that laughter lowered blood glucose levels in patients with type 2 diabetes by altering gene expression.

Even more exciting are the findings on the cardiovascular benefits of mirthful laughter. In a recent study by researchers at the University of Maryland, researchers found that endorphins released by the brain in response to laughter cause the production of nitric oxide (NO), which then triggers a number of cardio-protective signaling processes responsible for not only vasodilation but also for reducing platelet aggregation and vascular inflammation.

Laughter furthermore has been shown to have positive effects on the immune system. Professor Lee Berk from Loma Linda University reported that laughter increased the activity of several critical antibodies and natural killer cells, which are essential in anti-tumor defense. These studies represent only a small subset of the scientific literature attesting to the positive benefits of laughter.[1]

Cancer

For people living with cancer, it may seem strange to find humor when facing such serious issues. Yet, laughter may be helpful in ways you may not have realized or imagined.

Laughter may help you feel better about yourself and the world around you. Laughter may be a natural diversion. When you laugh, no other thought comes to mind. Laughing may also induce physical changes in the body. After laughing for only a few minutes, you may feel better for hours.

When used in addition to conventional cancer treatments, laughter therapy may help in the overall healing process.

Dr. Katherine Puckett, Chief of the Division of Mind-Body Medicine at Cancer Treatment Centers of America®, first introduced laughter therapy at our Illinois hospital upon a patient's request.

Laughter Club is based not on humor or jokes, but rather on laughter as a physical exercise. One group laughter exercise involves patients standing in a circle, with the leader in the middle. Patients put their fingertips on their cheekbones, chest or lower abdomen and make "ha ha" or "hee hee" sounds until they feel vibrations through their bodies. Dr. Puckett says that, during these exercises, it is hard for people not to join in because laughter is so contagious.

According to Dr. Puckett, at the end of a laughter therapy session, patients have said things like "I didn't even think about cancer during Laughter Club" and "That felt great! Things have been so hard that we hadn't laughed in months."[2]

Here's an email from a reader, who responded to an article I published about therapeutic laughter:

Dear Dr. Keith,

In 1968, my daughter, having just graduated with an honors degree in Microbiology, was diagnosed as having a Grade IV glioma.

We were all devastated as she was prepared for surgery.

One afternoon before she went into hospital, I sat in her room and read Roald Dahl's Revolting Rhymes. We both laughed until we cried!

Soon thereafter, I was in conversation with a homeopathic doctor, and I almost shamefully explained to him that we had laughed and laughed. Instead of admonishing us for being stupid, he told me that this was the best thing we could have done!

After surgery, the Neurosurgeon met with my wife and me and advised that we could expect to have our daughter for 9 months to 2 years because they had not been able to excise the tumor because it was too close to the brain stem. That's all he could offer.

It's a long story and our daughter experienced all the horrors of radiation 'therapy'. During this time, groups of us believers were in constant prayer, trusting God for a miracle.

In April 1969, the MRI scan showed that the tumor had disappeared. Gone!!!!

Now 28 years later, our daughter is married with a beautiful and talented daughter of her own.

When we hear of people being condemned to the 'cut, poison and burn' routine for their cancer therapy, we wonder why today's medicine men and women do not agree that chemo and radiation do not cure, and that alternative treatments (such as homoeopathy) should be used. And laughter, of course

Kind regards

I think this story is a reason, in and of itself, to laugh with an open heart!

Postscript: you might also want to check out Marci Schimoff's book *Happy For No Reason* (Free Press, New York, 2008).

Sources:

1. Can laughter be therapeutic. By Kaitlin McLean. http://www.yalescientific. org/2011/05/can-laughter-be-therapeutic/

2. http://www.cancercenter.com/treatments/laughter-therapy/

THE SIMONTONS

This is a famous name in cancer therapy, especially in respect of the power of the mind to heal effectively.

Dr. O. Carl Simonton MD (1942 - 2009) was an internationally acclaimed oncologist, author and speaker, best known for his pioneering insights and research in the field of psychosocial oncology. After earning a medical degree from University of Oregon Medical School, he completed a three-year residency in radiation oncology. During this time he developed his famous creative visualization approach for the treatment of cancer patients, the idea being that one's state of mind could influence one's ability to survive cancer.

Early in his medical career, Simonton noticed that patients given the same dose of radiation for similar cancers had different outcomes. When he looked into why, he concluded that people who had a more positive attitude generally lived longer and had fewer side effects.

His own research indicated that when lifestyle counseling was added to medical treatment for patients with advanced cancer, their survival time doubled and their quality of life improved.

A study by Stanford University and UC Berkeley researchers in 1989 concluded that women with advanced breast cancer who received emotional counseling lived about twice as long as those who did not.

The study was independent evidence that Simonton's "whole-body" approach to battling the illness made a difference, Dr. David Siegel, a psychiatrist and Stanford professor who wrote the study, wrote in an e-mail to The Times.

Simonton outlined his "will-to-live" philosophy of cancer care in *Getting Well Again*, a 1978 book written with his second wife, a psychotherapist then known as Stephanie Matthews-Simonton, and others.

The book was "highly praised" by officials at the National Institutes of Health and doctors who specialized in cancer and heart problems.

Thousands of counselors have been trained in the Simonton Method, which includes teaching patients to visualize their bodies fighting cancer cells -- and winning the war.

Talking openly about cancer was groundbreaking in the 1970s, as were such Simonton techniques as meditation and mental imagery. Today these approaches are open to anyone who has a mind to try them.

Here are the 10 main tenets of the Simonton approach, as published on the website of the Simonton Center in Santa Barbara:

1. Our emotions significantly influence health and recovery from disease (including cancer). Emotions are a strong driving force in the immune system and other healing systems.

2. Our beliefs and attitudes influence our emotions thereby affecting our health and healing systems.

3. We can significantly influence our beliefs and attitudes. As a result we shape our emotions, and therefore, significantly influence our health.

4. Ways of influencing beliefs, attitudes and emotions can be readily taught and learned by using a variety of accessible methods that are presented in this program.

5. All of us function as physical, mental, social and spiritual/philosophical beings. These aspects need to be addressed in the broad context of healing, with a focus on the particular needs of a person who is ill, and that person's family, community, and culture.

6. Harmony is central to health - balance among the physical, mental, and spiritual/philosophical aspects of being. This extends to relationships with self, family, friends, community, planet, and universe.

7. We have inherent (genetic, instinctual) tendencies and abilities that aid us in moving in the direction of health and harmony (physical, mental, spiritual/philosophical and social).

8. These abilities can be developed and implemented in meaningful ways through existing techniques and methods that are presented in this program.

9. As these abilities are developed, proficiency evolves, as when learning other skills. This results in greater harmony and improved quality of life, which significantly impacts one's state of health.

10. These skills and insights also change our relationship with death by lessening our fear and pain, and freeing more energy for getting well and living life more fully today.

[simontoncenter.com]

In November, 1997, Simonton was honored by the American Medical Association for his film, *Affirmations For Getting Well* by Touchstar Productions. This video, used in practically every hospital in the US, is presently being distributed to oncologists throughout the US by leading pharmaceutical giant GlaxoSmithKline.

Meanwhile, other researchers bitch and whine, "it's not proven."

Creative Visualizations

Consider this marvelous tale from the world of showbiz:

You may know David Seidler, who won an Oscar for best original screenplay for "The King's Speech," was a stutterer just like King George VI, whose battle with the speech disorder is portrayed in the 2010 film.

What you might not know is that Seidler, 73, suffered from cancer, just like the king did. But unlike his majesty, Seidler survived the cancer, and he says he did so because he used the same vivid imagination he employed to write his award-winning script.

Seidler says he visualized his cancer away.

"I know it sounds awfully Southern California and woo-woo," he admits when he describes the visualization techniques he used when his bladder cancer was diagnosed nearly six years ago. "But that's what happened."

Seidler says when he found out his cancer had returned, he visualized a "lovely, clean healthy bladder" for two weeks, and the cancer disappeared. He's been cancer-free for more than five years.

Whether you can imagine away cancer, or any other disease, has been hotly debated for years.

One camp of doctors will tell you that they've seen patients do it, and that a whole host of studies supports the mind-body connection. Other doctors, just as well-respected, will tell you the notion is preposterous, and there's not a single study to prove it really works.

Seidler isn't concerned about studies. He says all he knows is that for him, visualization worked.

"When I was first diagnosed in 2005, I was rather upset, of course," Seidler says in a telephone interview from his home in Malibu, California. "After three to four days of producing a lot of mucus and salty tears, I knew prolonged grief was bad for the *immune* system, and the *immune* system was the only buddy I had in fighting cancer." [my edit: Seidler used the term autoimmune system, which is somewhat misleading]

Seidler said that's when he decided to sit down and write the screenplay for "The King's Speech," which had been simmering in his brain for many years. "I thought, if I throw myself into the creative process, I can't be sitting around feeling sorry for myself," he says.

After consulting with California urologist Dr. Dino DeConcini, Seidler decided not to have chemotherapy or have all or part of his bladder removed, common treatments for bladder cancer. Instead, he opted for surgery to remove just the cancer itself, and he took supplements meant to enhance his immune system.

"For years, whenever I walked down the stairs I rattled like a pair of maracas, I had so many pills in me," he says.

Despite his best efforts, the cancer came back within months. Seidler was forced to rethink his decision not to have chemotherapy or bladder surgery.

At the suggestion of his then wife, Seidler decided to use the time while he waited for an operation to try to visualize his cancer disappearing.

"I spent hours visualizing a nice, cream-colored unblemished bladder lining, and then I went in for the operation, and a week later the doctor called me and his voice was very strange," Seidler said in an interview for CNN.

The doctor said, "I don't know how to explain it, but there's no cancer there." Seidler reports that the doctor was so confounded he sent the tissue from the presurgical biopsy to four different labs, and all confirmed they were cancerous.

Seidler says the doctor couldn't explain how it had happened. But Seidler believes the supplements and visualizations were behind his "spontaneous remission", plus a change in his way of thinking. He stopped feeling sorry for himself because of his cancer and his impending divorce.

"I was very grief-stricken," he remembers. "It was a 30-year marriage, and in my grief, I could tell I was getting sicker."

This is exactly in accord with Reike Geerd Hamer's "conflict-active" response—a tumor following a deeply wounding psychic shock. (see page 22)

"I decided to just change my head around," says Seidler.

While Seidler says he knows his unorthodox recovery techniques sound "woo-woo" to some ears, they sound "like science" to Dr. Christiane Northrup, a best-selling author who's written extensively on the mind-body connection.

"This doesn't sound woo-woo to me," she says. "The mind has the power to heal."

She says by moving himself "from fear and abject terror into action," Seidler changed his body's chemistry. "Fear increases cortisol and epinephrine in the body, which over time lower immunity," she says.

High levels of the two stress hormones lead to cellular inflammation, which is the way cancer begins, Northrup says. Taking action, as Seidler eventually did, decreases the hormones.

"Hope is actually a biochemical reaction in the body," she says.

Dr. Bernie Siegel, author of "Love, Medicine & Miracles," says it's the same way an athlete uses visualization to improve performance.

"When an athlete visualizes success, their body really is experiencing success. When you imagine something, your body really feels like it's happening," says Siegel, a retired clinical assistant professor of surgery at Yale Medical School.

In 1978 Siegel originated *Exceptional Cancer Patients*, a specific form of individual and group therapy utilizing patients' drawings, dreams, images and feelings. ECaP is based on "carefrontation," a safe, loving therapeutic confrontation, which facilitates personal lifestyle changes, personal empowerment and healing of the individual's life. The physical, spiritual and psychological benefits which followed led to his desire to make everyone aware of his or her healing potential. He realized exceptional behavior is what we are all capable of.

But Dr. Marcia Angell, former editor-in-chief of *The New England Journal of Medicine*, calls the mind-body connection a "new religion" that encourages false hope.

"There is something so biologically implausible that your attitude is going to cure a disease," says Angell, a senior lecturer in social medicine at Harvard Medical School. "There's a tremendous arrogance to imagine that your mind is all that powerful."

You are a tremendously arrogant (and ignorant) woman, Dr. Angell. We are not interested in your snotty opinion that something is "biologically implausible". "Experts" like you said anesthesia was biologically implausible... also antibiotics, heart transplants, kidney dialysis, pacemakers, driving a car at more than 30 miles an hour would explode the human frame, etc.

According to Angell, stories like Seidler's are just that -- only stories and not proof that the mind-body connection is real. But there was a time when putting someone to sleep and rendering them insensitive to pain while you amputated a leg was once "only a story."

Some other part of the patient's treatment plan likely explains success against the disease, or in other cases, the success is temporary and part of the natural course of the disease, Angell claims. Couldn't the same be said of orthodox chemotherapy: the apparency of a result is only a natural part of the cycle and chemo really does no good whatsoever?

Angell is trying to generalize from the fact that there are no large-scale studies showing visualization can treat disease, to the absurd claim that there is no proof that mind can influence health at all (even implying there is proof positive that this cannot happen, when such proof does NOT exist).

In fact the evidence points to the very opposite:

Vagus Nerve To The Rescue

Really, the naysayers' argument is destroyed by one simple scientific fact: measurement! There is no longer any room for mere opinion. Measurement of heart rate variability (HRV), which tells us how active the person's vagus nerve is, has been declared prognostic of cancer staging and progress.

The vagus nerve has what we call parasympathetic actions, meaning calming, relaxing and soothing (the opposite of flight or fight). High vagus activity means that cancer "staging" (stages I-IV) is less relevant and what's more cancer markers are significantly lower. Lower markers mean a less active tumor

Better still, vagal activity seems to protect against the ravages of cancer, by returning the body to homeostasis (balance). In homeostasis the patient won't feel so yuck and the body is in a more stable place from which to fight back against the disease.

In other words, recent studies have shown that *vagal nerve activity independently predicts prognosis in cancer.* [J Biol Regul Homeost Agents. 2014 Apr-Jun;28(2):195-201]

It's now beyond question that relaxed and favorable states of mind positively assist the fight against cancer. That means doctors who instill fear in their patients are being criminally unscientific, negligent and incompetent—a total disgrace to their profession.

The science of psychoneuroimmunology (PNI) is now fully established, whatever sneering Ms. Angell claims. [Vagal nerve activity predicts overall survival in metastatic pancreatic cancer, mediated by inflammation. Cancer Epidemiol. 2016 Feb;40:47-51. doi: 10.1016/j.canep.2015.11.007. Epub 2015 Nov 24]

A Visualization Guide

Whether you're convinced of the effects of visualization or not, Northrup says there's no harm in trying it, as long as you realize that like any other treatment, visualization might not work.

There's no definitive guide to visualization, but Siegel, who's instructed his patients in imaging for many years, has a few suggestions.

First, he says to draw a picture of four things: yourself, your health problem, your treatment and your body eliminating your problem. These pictures might tell you what sort of imagery would work best for you.

For example, when one of Siegel's patients drew her disease as 10 cancer cells next to one white blood cell, he suggested she visualize her body making more white blood cells.

Second, he says to know yourself. One religious patient of his had been visualizing dogs attacking and eating up her cancer, which didn't work, so instead she pictured her tumor as a block of ice and God's light melting it away, which he says was more effective.

Third, he suggests not visualizing anything violent, since most of us aren't violent by nature.

"Children don't mind being violent, and they'll visualize blasting away cancer, and that's fine, but most adults don't like to kill, so that's not an image they're comfortable with," he says. (see next section on electronic games)

He remembers one patient who was a Quaker and a pacifist, and quickly rejected any notion of "killing" or "beating" cancer. Instead, he pictured white blood cells carrying cancer cells away, and he beat his cancer.

[http://www.cnn.com/2011/HEALTH/03/03/ep.seidler.cancer.mind.body/]

My friend and mentor Dr. Patrick Kingsley used a similar metaphor of nurturing cancer cells, talking to them nicely and thinking of them as naughty children we want to persuade to behave. It's a good point to remind ourselves that cancer cells are not some alien beast dropped into our bodies from a flying saucer; they are simply normal cells gone wrong. As easily as they could turn bad, they could revert to normal again.

How Could This Work?

In interesting theory has been proposed as to how mental constructs of wellness could change real pathology in the tissues; it's called the "perception theory". The idea is that this is not really about transforming cognitive thoughts. But that the body's basic sensory apparatus in persuaded that there is a problem in how things are being perceived and this needs to be resolved. Consider the classic physiological experiment in which glasses are worn to invert the visual field. Eventually, after an interval, the brain makes changes that allow the visual field to be once ore seen as upright (if the glasses are then removed, the individual reverts to seeing things the "wrong way" up, though this was the original or "correct" orientation).

So with powerful visualizations, the basic brain apparatus is persuaded that something is wrong: there is a schema of disease and another imposed schema of health and wellbeing. One of the two must be wrong. The brain will adapt to make one of them true and the other loses out. When this works favorably, it means resolution has taken place towards the more healthy internal model.

In other words there is conflict resolution at a far more basic and subconscious level of mind function. I, for one, find this idea very persuasive.

The theory helps explain why certain illnesses may be more amenable to mind-body interaction, such as autoimmune conditions in which a sensory system (the immune system) has made an error. It also makes sense out of other healing modalities, such as those brought about by faith healers, shamans and "light workers", in which conflicts are resolved in favor of the "wrong" modality. [Psychon Bull Rev. 2012 Feb;19(1):24-45. doi: 10.3758/s13423-011-0166-x].

COMPUTER GAMES

If you really have a head for violence and fighting, some modern computer software games which depict the fight against cancer might appeal to you.

Notable is Re-Mission 2 (remission, get it?), a collection of six free online games—accessible via Web browsers or an Apple iPad—that share the theme of taking the fight to cancer. They do this by arming patients with a virtual arsenal of chemo, radiation and targeted cancer drug attacks designed to crush advancing malignant forces. The game—and its 2006 predecessor Re-Mission—are the product of HopeLab, a nonprofit founded in 2001 by Pamela Omidyar, wife of eBay founder Pierre Omidyar.

The six modules are: Nanobot's Revenge, Stem Cell Defender, Nano Dropbot, Leukemia, Feeding Frenzy and Special Ops.

It's hard to deny that a diversion such as "Stem Cell Defender," in which players protect white blood cells from a bacteria invasion by unleashing antibiotic bombs, could do wonders for a child's morale during long waits at a doctor's office or hospital. (Bacterial infections, nausea and constipation are some treatment-related effects patients may experience.) HopeLab, however, insists the games do even more than this, claiming they improve treatment outcomes by educating young patients about the disease and how it can be fought. Such knowledge makes these patients more likely to adhere closely to their treatment regimens.

Source: Scientific American blog: http://blogs.scientificamerican.com/observations/video-game-to-help-kids-fight-cancer/]

Ben's Wish

To my knowledge, this idea of software simulations of battling cancer first originated in 2004. A 9-year-old former leukemia patient Ben Duskin was asked if he had an unrequited wish by the Make-A-Wish Foundation. He requested a video game be made that fellow cancer sufferers could play to take their mind off the painful side effects of chemotherapy.

"I really like video games," Duskin said. "And I wanted to do something special, something more than going on a Disney cruise and stuff like that."

Enter Eric Johnston, a software engineer for LucasArts who helped create such games as "Indiana Jones and the Last Crusade," "Loom" and "The Secret of Monkey Island."

Johnston agreed to volunteer his time to help Ben achieve his wish. Johnston persuaded his bosses to donate LucasArts facilities after hours and met with Ben once a week for six months as they developed "Ben's Game."

The game's central character, modeled after Ben, zooms around the screen on a skateboard, zapping mutated cancer cells and collecting seven shields to protect against common side effects of chemotherapy, which include nausea, hair loss and fevers.

Duskin's leukemia is in remission. UCSF officials said "Ben's Game" is now a staple in the children's chemotherapy ward.

"I feel really good in my heart that lots of people are playing it," Ben said.

You Can Help Research Too

Scientists at Cancer Research UK have developed an intergalactic smartphone game to help them analyze the overwhelming reams of genetic data generated in recent studies. They hope thousands of people will play the game, simultaneously trawling through genetic material to pinpoint more precisely which genes cause the disease.

Using current DNA analysis techniques, scientists get readouts from tumor samples containing lots of peaks and troughs. And it's these highs and lows that are likely to harbor the genetic abnormalities they are looking for.

Computer software can help locate these to a certain extent, but the more precise judgment calls still need human eyes.

So game developers have transformed the readouts into an intergalactic landscape. It's called Play to Cure: Genes in Space. In the game, players navigate their spaceships safely around many obstructions while on a fast-paced mission to collect a precious material known as Element Alpha.

As they do so they guide their ships across mountains and valleys, corresponding to areas of the genome hiding the potentially cancer-promoting faults.

And as they travel through the landscape they trace a course that shows scientists the high and low bits - the bits where the mutations are likely to be.

The map each player plots is then sent back to scientists for interpretation. As more people highlight the peaks and troughs, scientists are alerted to these as areas worth further exploration.

The game draws on the largest genetic study into breast cancer, carried out in 2012, which changed the framework of how breast cancer is seen - from one broad disease into a disease of 10 different subtypes.

From the vast data gathered during this research, scientists search for areas of abnormalities known as copy number variations.

This is where sections of genetic material are either gained or lost - and these are known to be particularly important in the development of cancer.

Computer software is currently not accurate enough to do the job. In one in 10 cases something will be missed.

So researchers at Cancer Research UK and elsewhere are manually sifting through genetic material to detect the subtle changes that machines haven't yet been programmed to find.

By converting the data into a game, the charity hopes to harness the detection powers of thousands people, increasing the chance of specific genetic faults being found with accuracy and speed.

Prof Carlos Caldas, of Cancer Research UK, says: "Future cancer patients will be treated in a more targeted way based on their tumor's genetic fingerprint and our team is working hard to understand why some drugs work and others won't.

"But no device can do this reliably and it would take a long time to do the job manually. Play to Cure: Genes in Space will help us find ways to diagnose and treat cancer more precisely - sooner."

You can find Re-Mission 2 at: www.re-mission2.org

Join with Play To Cure: Genes In Space at: http://scienceblog.cancerresearchuk.org/2014/02/04/download-our-revolutionary-mobile-game-to-help-speed-up-cancer-research/

Ben's game can be downloaded for free at http://www.makewish.org/ben

And, of course, you are free to create any mental model you find works for you, with the theme of holding cancer in check, or destroying it. Let me call your attention to patient Tash's sheepdogs model, on page 37.

HELLINGER'S "FAMILY CONSTELLATIONS"

Most of our stress comes from family, if you think about it. Compared to the pressures they put us through, work, friends and even the government are relatively innocuous! Even if there is no malicious intent, loss, sickness, bereavement, etc. among our loved ones is one of the highest tolls on our wellbeing.

It may come as a surprise to you to know that family influences actually go back through the generations. Our grandparents and even our great grandparents can have a profound influence on our mental wellbeing. What your ancestors got up to, their struggles and strife—and their behavioral quirks and misdeeds even—can be a factor in the stress that led to you getting cancer, right now, today!

This is the life work of German psychotherapist Bert Hellinger. All cancer patients should know of his work and for many or most it would be a good idea to explore this dimension of healing and wellness.

Let me explain…

Bert Hellinger (b. 1925) spent 20 years as a Catholic priest, mostly in South Africa, also as a high school teacher and administrator, and missionary to the Zulu nation. After leaving the priesthood, he studied psychoanalysis, gestalt therapy, and transactional analysis. He is the author of some 30 books that have been translated into several languages. His "family constellations" therapeutic technique is popular throughout Europe, and has been growing into a worldwide phenomenon.

According to Hellinger, we have "unconscious connections with the fates of family ancestors" that must be revealed if psychotherapy is to be effective. Rupert Sheldrake's idea of morphic resonance could explain how we get "entangled" in the fates of our ancestors. "Fields of energy" have "memory and influence" that connect us in the present with people, places, and animals from the past. In short, Hellinger's "unconscious connections" are not genetic influences, nor are they repressed memories. They are thought of as psychic fields of energy.

The constantly surprising findings, particularly in quantum physics, brings science ever closer to spirituality, i.e. the consciousness of our deep interconnectedness and of love being our original quality and our essence. Quantum physics and spirituality are teaching us that we are deeply connected ("entangled" in quantum language) to all and everything: what happens to others happens equally to us in a very concrete way.

One of Hellinger's early influences was family therapist Virginia Satir, who introduced us to family conjoint therapy. What she found was that if you consider the family as a whole dynamic structure, medicine changes. If you successfully treat a schizophrenic, very often someone else in the family will develop schizophrenia (psychiatrists slide over this inconvenient fact rather easily). You need to treat the entire family.

It may be the same with cancer, according to Hellinger's theory: the family energy dynamic calls forth a cancer and someone has to get it. Obviously, then, we want to re-structure the entire family constellation, otherwise another member of the family may similarly fall ill.

In setting up a family constellation at a workshop, a client chooses work-shop attendees to represent members of his or her family, then places them in relationship to each other, without comment, based on how it "felt" to be in the family. Despite not knowing each other or having much information about the family members or their relationships to each other, the representatives become a living model of the original family system.

This may sound weird but I have attended a Hellinger workshop, run by the big man himself. The subject had throat cancer and was struggling to come to terms with the full meaning of her life. He put people hither and thither in the room, based on intuition and feelings. Then, as soon as the constellation depicted reached a certain shape, 90% of the audience (me included) burst into tears. The emotion in the room was powerful, palpable and inescapable.

In fact full-size "representatives" are not required. They may be substituted by small figures moved about on a tabletop, sheets of paper or footprints placed on the floor, the therapist standing in for family members, or the client him- or herself moving from place to place. The constellation may even be done in the form of a guided visualization that the client experiences with eyes closed or in the form of a story told by the facilitator.

According to Hellinger, the therapy begins by having the client state what the problem is and what outcome he or she is looking for. The kinds of problems he cites as being a result of energy entanglements are: "feelings of isolation, depression, mental and physical illness, accidents, financial or relationship issues, and even suicidal thoughts or attempts." Through the use of the morphic field, "entanglements may be seen, unresolved issues may be addressed, and resolutions may be found which release the flow of love in your life."

Or, as Hellinger's mentor Dr. Albrecht Mahr—a medical doctor, a specialist in mind-body medicine and systems therapy—puts it:

We are inflicting on ourselves what we reject, fight, and destroy. And the practice of compassion, loving kindness, and perceiving the human being in the opponent are the intelligent expression of our very own self-interest.

Will Hellinger's method work for you? The only way to find out is to try it. I have to add the caveat, as with all such things, *that it depends to a great extent on the skill of the facilitator and not so much on the validity of Hellinger's theories*.

Journalist Florian Burkhardt reports on participating in a family constellation session:

As an observing, though skeptical journalist, I also agreed to enter several constellations during the workshop. Some of the feelings that I had during those constellations were not my own, and I cannot explain their origin. It felt as if you could tune on a TV set and watch your deepest family relations unfold, with the therapist holding the remote control.

Burkhardt's additional observation is worth noting:

How this knowing field comes to exist has always been a secret (even to me) and its existence has never been scientifically proven. Experts say that the concept of "knowing fields" has most likely developed out of tribal rituals in South Africa, where Mr. Bert Hellinger, the German founder of the therapy movement, spent some time as a Catholic missionary.

Of course there are critics who knock this. Positive outcomes from the therapy have been attributed to conventional explanations such as suggestion and empathy but without a shred of evidence to support this off-the-wall contempt. [Robert T. Carroll at skepdic.com]

A Word Of Warning: ignore Hellinger's set theories about incest, homosexuality and so on. These are just a distraction. So is the fact that many Hellinger practitioner turncoats distanced themselves from their founder, as a result of a poem by Hellinger, directed to Hitler, telling him he was not inhuman but just as vulnerable as the rest of us.

"I look upon you as I look upon myself: namely as a human being with a father and a mother, and with an extraordinary fate... If I respect you, then I respect myself. And if I loathe you, then I loathe myself."

Personally, if I were looking for a good practitioner, I would avoid anyone who rejects Hellinger because of this poem. That person know *nothing* about humanity, soul and compassion. It is vital to the workings of family constellations that nothing is excluded on the grounds of politically-correct dogma.

Read again the words of Albrecht Mahr above.

THE RELAXATION RESPONSE

You might think this topic has only indirect connection to states of mind. You would be wrong. Herbert Benson's "Relaxation Response" is crucial to how we think, feel and act. It's a sort of meditative physiology, without the oriental mystery and pseudo-religious beliefs that seem to get attached to meditation.

The Relaxation response is actually the direct opposite of the familiar "fight or flight" of urgent physiological changes that leap into action when a creature senses danger. First described by Walter Bradford Cannon over 80 years ago, this model states that animals react to threats with a general discharge of the sympathetic nervous system, preparing the animal for fighting or running away. More specifically, the adrenal glands produce a cascade of hormones, notably adrenalin and noradrenalin (norepinephrine and epinephrine). Later cortisol, which is very damaging, enters the picture when stress becomes chronic.

The Relaxation Response, on the other hand, is characterized by eat, sleep and chill. It's a mental, physical and emotional response leading to a place of deep rest.

Herbert Benson, a Harvard University cardiologist, distinguished himself by demonstrating, scientifically (with instruments and recordings), that there is no magic or transcendental mystery to the Maharishi's Transcendental Meditation ™

That in fact there is no need for a mantra or chanting "Om". Just repeating a simple word, or even just the number "One", over and over, has identical effects... and it's free! Catholics might want to try the "Hail Mary" prayer. Just keep it simple, stupid (K.I.S.S.)

Here are the steps, following instructions in *The Relaxation Response*, pages 162-163:

1. Sit quietly in a comfortable position (don't lie down, this is not sleep).

2. Close your eyes.

3. Deeply relax all your muscles, beginning at your feet and progressing up to your face. Keep everything relaxed.

4.   Breathe gently through your nose. Become aware of your breathing. As you breathe out, say your chosen word or just "one", silently to yourself. For example, breathe in ... out, "one",- in ... out, "one", etc. Breathe easily and naturally.

5.   Do this for 10 to 20 minutes, once or twice a day but at least once. You may open your eyes to check the time, but do not use an alarm. When you finish, sit quietly for several minutes, at first with your eyes closed and then with your eyes opened.

6.   If you can't sit still that long, do it while you are exercizing. Say your word on each foot fall if you're running, or with each stroke if you are swimming.

Don't even worry about whether you are successful in achieving a deep level of relaxation. Maintain a passive attitude and just let relaxation come at its own pace. When distracting thoughts occur, that's not a failure either. Just try to ignore them by not dwelling upon them and return to repeating your word, phrase or "one."

Don't try this within two hours of a meal, since the digestive processes seem to interfere with the elicitation of the Relaxation Response.

With practice, the response should come with little effort.

Don't get involved with mantras. It's better to use a soothing, gentle sound, preferably with no meaning, or association, to avoid stimulation of unnecessary thoughts.

As Benson says, it's hard for people to accept this simple technique: "It's so easy. The main problem we're having now in this context is its simplicity. Our culture feels that unless something is expensive, mechanical, complicated, it must not work. But if you make it more complicated you destroy its essence, which is passivity and simplicity." [Interview with *The Washington Post*]

There are scores of other ways to summon the relaxation response, as well, said Benson at the American Psychological Association's 2008 address. "Anything that breaks the train of everyday thought will evoke this physiological state."

That includes participating in repetitive sports such as running, letting go of tension through progressive muscular relaxation, practicing yoga, knitting, crocheting, even playing musical instruments.

"You know how when you play an instrument and you become 'one' with that instrument and the time flits away? That is the relaxation response," he said. "You know the high you get from running? That is the relaxation response coming about by the repetitive motion of your footfall."

Rest and Sleep

And while we are now on the subject of simplicity and relaxation, let's look at sleep.

Without question, proper sleep is one of the most healing and restorative physiological tools we have to overcome disease. Sleep deprivation does the opposite. According to the "Sleep Doctor" Micheal Breus, the more sleep deprived you are, the faster cancer cells grow!

Michael Irwin investigated the effect of disturbed sleep patterns in depressed patients and found a positive correlation between poor sleep patterns and reduced NK cell activity in both the depressed and control subjects. The specific functions of sleep are not known, although sleep is commonly considered a restorative process that is important for the proper functioning of the immune system. Severity of disordered sleep in depressed and alcoholic subjects correlates with declines in natural and cellular immunity and is associated with alterations in the complex cytokine network.

By now you will know that lowered immune function is a significant risk factor for developing cancer and having a lowered ability to fight it, once you have got it. *So we conclude that deep and restful sleep is a crucial factor in the psychology of fighting cancer.*

[Neuropsychopharmacology (2001) 25, S45–S49. doi:10.1016/S0893-133X(01)00338-4]

Sleep is traditionally divided into "sleep cycles" of about 90 minutes each. There are four stages of sleep and we cycle through each. Stages 1 and 2 are REM sleep, so-called (from random eye movements, which characterize that level of sleep).

In the US, stages 3 and 4 are combined to form what is lumped together as "deep sleep". In the rest of the world, the stage 3 and 4 terminology is used. It takes a full cycle to go down from stages 1 and 2, to deep sleep, and back up. There are five sleep cycles per night (making a total of 7 ½ hours, rather than 8 hours).

What we do know is that the first sleep cycle (before midnight) is about restoration and repair. The later cycles have to do with processing short-term memory and converting it to long-term.

Conclusion? You need to be in bed well before midnight and fast asleep. 10.30 is a good bedtime for those battling cancer. It's good for the rest of us, too!

Study the chart below: you'll see that the first two sleep cycles are quite deep. After that they become shallower.

A Typical 8 Hour Sleep Cycle

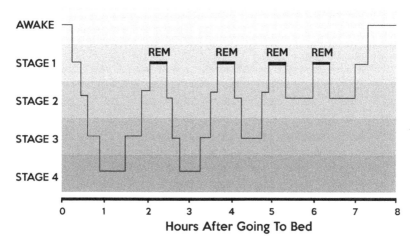

Hours After Going To Bed

FLOWER REMEDIES TO ADJUST PSYCHOLOGY

Here's a strange thing, if you haven't already met it: the idea that flower "essences" can adjust your thinking and help you through tough times.

It goes back to an English physician (OK, with a Welsh name) who developed a new discipline. Dr. Edward Bach (pronounced like batch) was a homeopath and is rightly famous for the development of a number of bowel "nosodes" (a nosode is a homeopathic preparation made from obnoxious or toxic materials, such as bacteria, designed to dislodge a condition within the body).

But he was perhaps not so comfortable using remedies derived from hostile sources. He wanted something purer, gentler and simpler. He eventually hit on the idea of flower essences.

Like any good physician, Dr. Bach knew that attitude of mind plays a vital role in maintaining health and recovering from illness. After identifying 38 basic negative states of mind and spending several years exploring the countryside, he managed to create a plant or flower based remedy for each one.

Bach was what we would call a "sensitive", he touched flowers and he got vibrations or "messages", as to what the plant would heal. It all sounds a bit woo-woo but there is no question: Bach's flower remedies work and work well.

Wanting to make his flower essences more available to the general public, Bach enlisted the help of Nelsons Homeopathic Pharmacy in London back in the 1930s. Under his instruction, they began to make and sell stock remedies from the mother tinctures he supplied. In 1990, this relationship was formalized, and since then Nelsons (the Pharmacy's parent company) has been responsible for all the bottling and distribution of the Bach remedies.

Today, Nelsons produces millions of stock bottles each year from its warehouse facility in Wimbledon, London, and the Bach® Original Flower Remedies are sold in over 70 countries around the world.

His premier formulation, called "Rescue remedy" (made from Cherry Plum, Clematis, Impatiens, Rock Rose and Star of Bethlehem) should be on every medicine cupboard. It can be obtained from virtually any pharmacy and whole food store. It's good for shock, trauma, fear, panic, tension and mood changes.

The original Bach natural remedies have been used confidently in Europe for over 100 years. If you like celebrity endorsements, Jennifer Aniston says it keeps her cool under pressure; Cate Blanchett and Salma Hayek have been fans for years; Roberta Flack uses the soothing effect of "Rescue Remedy®" for menopausal hot flashes.

There's also a sleep formulation, with added white chestnut. See page 82 on why sound sleep is a very important part of fighting cancer:

White Chestnut: To help ease restless mind.

Star of Bethlehem: For trauma and shock.

Clematis: For the tendency to "pass out", and unconsciousness, being 'far away' and not present mentally.

Cherry Plum: Fear of mind giving way, verge of breakdown, anger.

Impatiens: For irritability, tension and fidgetiness.

Rock Rose: For frozen terror and panic.

Flower essences have proved to be of great help in restoring "the will to live," overcoming the shadow of this extreme diagnosis, giving strength to the organism and helping the patient to respond positively towards any chosen treatment regimen, by altering the mental landscape. Flower essences can bring optimism, courage, determination and strength.

As Dr. Marina Angeli, a psychiatrist in Athens, Greece, put it: Flower essences have proven to be very important [to a cancer case] in cleansing and rebalancing mental-emotional states, giving space to the person's soul to bring him/her back to life again, by unblocking the energy system to a point where it is able to nourish and cure the body.

Please note: this is not the same as saying flower essences themselves may in any way effect a cure. Only nature and the mental determination of the patient can do that. But flower essences may also help to mitigate the unpleasant side-effects of heavy treatment regimens, such as chemo or radio-therapy, if the patient has opted for the orthodox path.

There are books on flower remedies, which give far more detail on the actions of each of Bach's remedies that I can manage here. Suffice it to mention:

Olive

Bach described Olive as the remedy for "those who have suffered much mentally or physically and are so exhausted and weary that they feel they have no more strength to make any effort." The remedy helps to restore enthusiasm for life. It helps you tap into a higher source and thereby find new energy and restoration at all levels.

Elm

Elm is for those who "suddenly feel overwhelmed by their responsibilities and feel inadequate to deal with them or keep up with events; this is often brought about by taking on too much work without taking care of oneself. As a result they feel depressed and exhausted, with a temporary loss of self-esteem." The remedy helps you find balance in your life, setting realistic expectations and goals. It also helps you to be open to receiving assistance from others and from the Higher Self.

Walnut

Walnut is a remedy specifically to help in dealing with change of any sort: divorce, marriage, change in career, menopause, or any change in circumstances. Some workers use Walnut for dealing with jet lag and what I call "travel shock" (the general effects of moving from country to country). Anyone who has been diagnosed with cancer is already facing a major change in life. Walnut can help you navigate through change in a positive way, following your inner direction, while at the same time protecting you from negative external influences.

Mimulus

Mimulus brings courage in the face of known and understandable fears, such as flying, a hospital visit, a confrontation over some unpleasantness in the family, or an illness, such as cancer. Those with marked Mimulus traits tend to be physically delicate and wilting, with a tendency to blush easily, stammer, or suddenly become speechless. Others talk too much from sheer nervousness.

Other Flower Remedies

It only remains to mention there are other flower essence ranges. But I have no experience of these and so am unable to make comparison or recommendations.

Ones that you may come across include The Ranger Of Light essences, the Findhorn range, Himalayan Flower Enhancers and Australian Bush Flower Essences (which distributes *mulla-mulla*, good for fighting off radiation sickness (see page 37).

If you want to learn more about flower essences, I suggest you start with Edward Bach, "The Twelve Healers," in *The Bach Flower Remedies* (New Canaan, Conn.: Keats Pub., 1997).

MEASURING HAPPINESS AND BALANCE

Happiness is a very ephemeral hard-to-understand phenomenon; we just like how it feels. But what is going on in our bodies when we get that nice, warm, fuzzy feeling?

The secret is what we call the autonomic nervous system (autonomic: it runs itself, silently, without our knowing). This aspect of our brain and neural networks is divided into two contrasted parts: the sympathetic nervous system and the parasympathetic nervous system. These are complementary to each other: where one fires you up, the other calms you down. They work together. They must be in harmony for you to enjoy optimum health.

I'm talking now about the vital health principle of balance.

Too much *yang* energy and not enough *yin* energy is bad; too much acid and not enough alkali is bad (and in the reverse); too much exercise and not enough rest and sleep is bad; too much excitement and not enough calm and recovery time is bad... we need B-A-L-A-N-C-E.

But because we are living such pressurized lives in a fragmented, buzz-fed world, what tends to happen is that we go over the top with sympathetic stimulation. That means adrenalin, fast heart, tension and excitement. It's exciting living on the edge for a time but we can't keep this up; it would be exhausting, unhealthy and, eventually, wreck our bodies.

The missing element is the parasympathetic tone to balance this. The parasympathetic system calms everything down—it slows the heart and breathing, lowers blood pressure and reduces inflammation.

The principal parasympathetic nerve, the vagus, visits almost every organ in the body, bringing the soothing signals of quiet and calm. In fact it has been discovered that vagus nerve stimulation is brilliant at settling down inflammation. Already vagus nerve stimulation is being used to quell arthritis, stop autoimmune diseases and reduce painful irritation, caused by inflammation. Don't forget, cancer has a strong inflammatory component too.

Parasympathetic is gentler and potentially healing, whereas sympathetic tone is not. Thus balance in our autonomic function, especially enough relax-recovery-parasympathetic time, is important to all aspects of health and even how long we live. According to the American Journal of Cardiology, "...healthy longevity depends on preservation of autonomic function, in particular, parasympathetic function represents a marker predictive of longevity."

[The American Journal of Cardiology, 2010 Apr 15; 105(8): 1181-5]

How Do We Know What's Happening?

Thing is, how do we measure this? Most people have lost the ability to feel what autonomic state they are in. Modern living has us very much out of tune with our bodies.

Actually there is a surprisingly simple and easy way to measure autonomic tone and that's monitoring heart rate variability (HRV). For the longest time, doctors and scientists believed that heart rate was constant, or should be—a monotonous regular frequency was considered "healthy".

As with so many things that were once "scientific fact", this turned out to be nonsense. The truth is 180 degrees round: marked variability is now known to be the healthy finding.

In general, a high HRV indicates dominance of the parasympathetic response, the side of the autonomic nervous system I have explained promotes relaxation, digestion, sleep, and recovery. The parasympathetic system is also known as the "eat, sleep and digest" system. It's what you (and lions) do after a heavy meal.

A low HRV indicates dominance of the sympathetic response, the fight or flight side of the nervous system associated with stress, slow recovery and inflammation. It's characterized by the secretion of adrenalin and cortisol, both high stress hormones.

Studies have made it clear that HRV is significantly lower in cancer patients than the healthy population [M. de Couck and Y. Gidron, "Norms of vagus nerve activity, indexed by heart rate variability, in cancer patients," *Cancer Epidemiology*, vol. 37, no. 5, pp. 737–741, 2013] and decreased HRV was associated with significantly shorter survival rates in cancer patients [N. Fadul, F. Strasser, J. L. Palmer et al., "The association between autonomic dysfunction and survival in male patients with advanced cancer: a preliminary report," *Journal of Pain and Symptom Management*, vol. 39, no. 2, pp. 283–290, 2010].

You can monitor your HRV using a simple smartphone app. I have the SweetBeat app (www.sweetwaterhrv.com) and recommend that (it's about $10). You can shop around for your own. You will also need a heart rate monitor; the kind that straps to your chest is the most accurate but you can use wristbands. Polar do a bluetooth version for $50, available on Amazon.

Again, you can shop for your own (just make sure the monitor is compatible with the phone app).

I recommend that everyone with cancer get an HRV monitor system and get that number up, or if your system measures balance, get it to 1:1. If there is one single measurement that tells most accurately the general state of your health, it's HRV. **This backs up my entire book: NOTHING is more important for your health, wellbeing and lifespan than keeping your heart rate flexible and changing.**

The bottom line is this: <u>studies have demonstrated repeatedly that autonomic dysfunction is associated with shorter survival in patients with advanced cancer</u>. Here's just one example: a study from the *Journal of Clinical Neurology* (Dec 2015) Their conclusion was brutal but simple: the presence of cancer in combination with decreased heart rate variability is associated with shorter survival time. [Prognostic Value of Heart Rate Variability in Patients With Cancer. J *Clin Neurophysiol*. 2015 Dec;32(6):516-20. doi: 10.1097/WNP.0000000000000210.]

Cardiologists and other cardiac specialists have been using HRV for decades to track the health and recovery of their patients, and it's why HRV is a predictive indicator of overall heart health, risk of heart attack, and other cardiac events.

Among the elderly, a high HRV is strongly associated with living long and living well; the kind of graceful aging relatively free of morbidity we all desire.

It should be around 78 – 80. Typical is 60 – 65. If it's below 50, that means you have a massive uphill struggle to battle against any disease, never mind cancer.

You need to take your HRV reading at the same time each day (in the morning is best). Trends over time are more important than individual readings. Individual low results are nothing to worry about. Lack of sleep, stress or a sore throat can drive down your measurements.

So How Do We Get A Better HRV?

Basically, anything which calms and relaxes you is good for your HRV. Turning off the TV, massage, quality time with your loved ones, gentle music, an absorbing hobby... all these help our wellbeing.

- Set aside time in nature, walk barefoot outside, turn off your smart-phone, unplug from technology.

- Sleep quality and quantity is crucial. I have already outlined this on page 82.

- All good health measures work. Remember by maxim: ALL GOOD HEALTH MEASURES ARE ANTI-CANCER MEASURES. You don't need weird and over-sold solutions to cancer; even holistic remedies—not even oxygen, enzymes and supplements—so much as you need the basics of sound physiology, as outlined in this section.

- Try getting cold on purpose: take a cold shower, cold bath, cold swim, you could try cryotherapy (supposed to release endorphins, which are hormones that make you feel good and energetic. The mood-enhancing effects from each session can last for days).

- Do a frequent parasympathetic reset (Tahiti Pose) – Insight, Denneroll

- Yoga, meditation, dance and movement! These are all good ways to work on improving your HRV.

Guided Imagery

A number of studies have shown that HRV can be significantly improved by guided imagery training [BioMed Research International. Volume 2015 (2015), Article ID 687020, 8 pages. http://dx.doi.org/10.1155/2015/687020].

One of the great ways to do this is by using modern devices that are capable of brain entrainment. An important study published in 2013 found a significant relationship between alpha brainwave entrainment and HRV.

Each of ten subjects, 4 males and 6 females, listened to 20 minutes of alpha stimulation (at 8 – 10 Hz), generated by a Neuro-Programmer device.

The research team then compared the average total HRV experienced by subjects during the at rest state to that experienced during the alpha stimulation, and noted an increase for each subject in total variability, ranging from a 20% to a 68% improvement.

[World Journal of Neuroscience, 2013, 3, 213-220 WJNS http://dx.doi.org/10.4236/wjns.2013.34028]

My own modality of Multi-Media Sensory Stimulation (MMSS) combines brain entrainment using binaural beats, with photic driving (light), slow de-stimulating music, coupled with creative "mind walks"!

There are a number of devices on the market, capable of creating brain entrainment through binaural beats, photic driving, music and creative voice imagery.

My favorite at this time is the Kasina, from Robert Austin's Mind Place (www.mindplace.com). Kasina is a Sanskrit (actually Pali) word which refers to an ancient system of meditation that uses visual objects to focus the mind.

The Kasina has perfect build quality and its presentation (unboxing as the Americans say) is very attractive.

There is a built-in an MP3 player and an 8 GB microSD card included, with over 50 audio-visual excursions, with aural backgrounds ranging from the soothing sounds of nature to ambient electronic tapestries to embedded binaural beats and isochronic pulses-all beautifully orchestrated and synchronized to the visual experience.

You can also listen to tracks by me, particularly a white light meditation, which you should find helpful for mastering any kind of pain.

The Kasina also features a backlit, colored LCD display, a built in rechargeable lithium battery, and can be used as a USB external audio device. It's also the most capable AudioStrobe decoder on the market, with 16 different color-mapping presets. Use the Color Organ feature to turn any music into a colorful light show-and it includes six different settings, to help match the mood of your music. And the GanzFrames (glasses) feature six colored LEDs per eye, for an even more intense experience, should you desire.

What I like especially is that you are not tied to tracks only from the Mind Place website. You can load any mp3 of your own choosing. You can put your playlists up there! The Kasina includes a free editor app for both Mac and Windows, on the included flash memory card.

Imagine a world of pure, jewel-like color illuminating your visual and mental fields. Amazing visual effects can be produced, including the illusion of complex, shifting geometrical patterns. This imagery, in combination with soothing, flowing sounds, can be so compelling that the mind clears of extraneous thoughts. In this way the Kasina experience is a form of meditation that is highly beneficial for cancer sufferers.

It's also great for reducing perceptions of pain, by the way, which I know can be an issue for cancer sufferers.

Neuropeptides

How do these amazing mental and emotional changes take place? Many researchers believe different brain wave patterns are linked to the production in the brain of various neuropeptides associated with relaxation and stress release. These neuropeptides include beta-endorphins, acetylcholine, vaso-pressin, and serotonin.

Dr. Margaret Patterson in collaboration with biochemist Dr. Ifor Capel at the Marie Curie Cancer Memorial Foundation Research Department in Surrey, England, has shown that certain frequencies in the brain dramatically speed up production of a variety of neurotransmitters, different frequencies triggering different brain chemicals. For instance, a 10 Hz (alpha) signal boosts the production and turnover rate of serotonin, a chemical messenger that increases relaxation and eases pain, while catecholamines, vital for memory and learning, respond at around 4 Hz (theta).

Dr. William Bauer, one of the foremost experts in the field of electromedicine, tells us more: "What I think is happening...is that by sending out the proper frequency, proper waveform and proper current...we tend to change the configuration of the cell membrane...Cells that are at sub-optimal levels are stimulated to 'turn on' and produce what they're supposed to produce, probably through DNA, which is stimulated through the cell membrane... You're charging the cells through a biochemical process that can possibly balance the acetylcholine or whatever neurotransmitter needs to be turned on..." [Harvey, Ruth S. The Miracle of Electromedicine. National Institute of Electromedical Information, Inc. digest Bulletin, Winter, 1985].

By now readers will know that anything which restores cell potential and normalcy is likely to benefit cancer sufferers.

PART 3

WHAT CANCER CAN TEACH US

No need to wait till your cancer has gone before we look beyond it. Here's a great question for you to think about:

If your cancer were whisked away magically (and completely) tomorrow, what changes would you bring into your life?

It's a trick question, in a way. Because if you DON'T make significant changes, it could show up again. You need to look beyond the "bad luck" model and, having read this far and figured out many of the potential trigger factors you have been carrying around, you need to eradicate them. Create a whole new life, starting now...

The passive patient who says just, "The doctors have cured me. They told me there was no trace of cancer any more," is playing with fire. Not to make changes is taking an enormous and unjustifiable risk.

There were causes for your disease and, just because doctors are trained (yes, trained) to ignore these causes, so he or she will have done little to take you through the modifiable risk factors. Indeed, many doctors seem to think there are no modifiable risk factors. It's all "in your genes" and after that it's just a question of random chance—whether you get cancer or, if you have got it, whether you are one of the unlucky ones who won't make it.

This is contrary to all of today's science. But it's a dogma deeply embedded in medico-politics.

UNCONDITIONAL LOVE

It's a word or phrase you read often. But what is it? Does it have any meaning, really?

Here are some fine words from Bernie Siegel MD, from an interview by his wife, Barbara H. Siegel, posted at The Well Being Journal (https://www.well-beingjournal.com):

"The illness gives me a chance to teach people about unconditional love: giving with no expectations because one chooses to give. Discipline and saying no are permitted between two people sharing this love. It is the conditional love upon which most of us are brought up that leads to illness. We never get all the "thank yous" and praise we would like. It is having something to give that restores us and provides us with a reason for living, when what we are giving is unconditional love. Physical handicap or illness does not interfere with the ability to give love. Invariably the love is returned to us without our asking, because people see the change and want to be closer to this new found peace.

"Many of my patients who are physically quite ill, some near death, wonder why they still have so many visitors. I explain to them that their spirit is very much alive and that "terminal" is a state of mind. Their spirit and love attract others because the others see life, not death, and therefore are comfortable in their presence."

In 1926 Elida Evans, in her book entitled *A Psychological Study of Cancer*, said, "Cancer is a symbol, as most illness is, of something going wrong in the patient's life, a warning to him to take another road." Those who take this new road find a new life, exceed expectations and sometimes are cured of incurable illness. The new lifestyle is the goal, not physical well-being. The latter is the traditional medical approach.

Physician as a Spiritual Teacher

The physician can be a spiritual leader and help people be reborn, Siegel says. Patients are usually not upset with the doctor for not healing them physically, but they actually thank him or her for the new life and ability to love. They feel this way because they have been made eternal in the only way possible...

"The secret to being eternal is love. Thornton Wilder said, "And we ourselves shall be loved for a while and then forgotten, but the love will have been enough, even memory is not necessary for love. There is a land of the dead, and the bridge is love." It can be said in another way: to die, but not to perish, that is eternity. Love teaches us how not to perish.

"There is eternal life through love, yet part of the reason physicians have no need to deal with this problem is that unconsciously they believe doctors don't get sick or die. (This is an unconscious reason for many to become doctors, but it is never addressed during medical training. There is a massive denial that keeps them from feeling what their patients feel and, therefore, from needing to face illness and death)."

I must say, I don't recognize myself in this. But it's an interesting take on becoming a doctor!

"One patient, when confronted with a dismal future leading to the grave, asked her doctor (who made the prognosis), "But what can I do?" He replied, "You only have a hope and a prayer." She asked, "How do I hope and pray?" And he said, "I don't know, that's not my line of work." With my help she has learned to hope and pray. She has transcended her physical illness and her fears, and now she goes to her doctor to bring him life and love. He, inciden-tally, has become very busy making notes about her exceptional course."

SEARCHING FOR THE POSITIVE

Here's a cheerful life hack that will see what positive changes have *already* come into your life, as a result of the cancer. Yes, you read that right. I did say positive changes that may have come about because of your cancer.

It's from Dr. John Demartini's lead. He asks you to consider your life in sev-en (7) key zones: mental, finances, vocation, spirituality, social connections, physical health and, last but not least, family.

Get yourself a notepad (this is like journaling). Ask yourself this key question:

In [that life zone] what positive thing has come into my life, as a result of my cancer diagnosis?

Don't be skeptical. There should be plenty to write about in each zone. Many patients, indeed, say that cancer produced profound and positive changes in their life, from getting rid of the negative, eliminating unimportant and time-wasting activities, discovering new bonds of love and friendship that became more precious than ever, to starting to be serious about health issues, taking control of diet and exercize programs, and working through issues which had long been ignored.

Patients report such positives as feeling more alive, getting to spend more time with family members, feeling supported when friends visit or send gifts, feeling a deeper love with more meaning, letting go of the trivial and focusing on what you DO have, instead of what you don't have in life.

One of the recurring positives is being able to take control of emotions and feelings and react more intelligently to what life throws at you, ensuring that you live that day and every day, with full engagement.

One woman expressed it this way: "Cancer wrecked my body—and thankfully my inhibitions. I'm no longer afraid to hug a stranger, hold a friend's hand, or say "I love you"!" (http://www.healthcentral.com/breast-cancer/c/78/180622/ve-cancer-survivors-speak/)

In October 2014, *Cosmopolitan Magazine*, no less, ran an article entitled: "How cancer changed my life... for the better":

One woman reported she began to appreciate every single day; that every moment counts; not a day goes by when I am not grateful for this experience, she said. It even focused her on true love and she married the man of her desires, instead of waiting.

Another woman was diagnosed with Hodgkin's Lymphoma. She wanted to travel the world and went to South East Asia, Australia and California among other places. It was incredible. "So many times in life," her words, "You want to do something but there's an always an excuse that gives you a reason to put it off. But when you have cancer, you HAVE to seize the moment, you run out of excuses."

The great physician-writer-philosopher Oliver Sacks learned he was sure to die of cancer (it had taken serious hold of his liver). But even then, there were plenty of positives to revel in:

Over the last few days, I have been able to see my life as from a great altitude, as a sort of landscape, and with a deepening sense of the connection of all its parts. This does not mean I am finished with life.

On the contrary, I feel intensely alive, and I want and hope in the time that remains to deepen my friendships, to say farewell to those I love, to write more, to travel if I have the strength, to achieve new levels of understanding and insight.

This will involve audacity, clarity and plain speaking; trying to straighten my accounts with the world. But there will be time, too, for some fun (and even some silliness, as well).

I feel a sudden clear focus and perspective. There is no time for anything inessential. I must focus on myself, my work and my friends. I shall no longer look at "NewsHour" every night. I shall no longer pay any attention to politics or arguments about global warming...

I cannot pretend I am without fear. But my predominant feeling is one of gratitude. I have loved and been loved; I have been given much and I have given something in return; I have read and traveled and thought and written. I have had an intercourse with the world, the special intercourse of writers and readers.

People who are older when they are diagnosed with cancer tend to find more growth or benefits after the experience. This may be because, as you get older, your ability to think about complex ideas grows, and the idea of finding something beneficial in having a life-threatening disease like cancer is complex. Also, people who are older when they are diagnosed with cancer may be more involved in treatment decisions and think more deeply about the impact of cancer and its treatment, including both positive and negative aspects.

People who are more optimistic in general also tend to see greater benefits from having cancer. This suggests that the way you look at life in general is similar to the way you look at your cancer experience. If you tend to look on the bright side of things most of the time, you may also have an easier time looking for the positives in having cancer.

20 Reasons To Be Glad You Got Cancer

Blogger Steven Eddy actually went so far as to create a list of "Top 20 Reasons Why I'm Glad I Got Cancer" (FYI, he did not have to think very hard about these...Steven says he banged out a rough list of 20 reasons in less than 10 minutes! (https://steveneddy.wordpress.com)

Here are his first 10, which you may find helpful when looking for your own positives:

1) Extra time with my wife; although my numerous medical appointments are a big time commitment, it does mean 2 or 3 extra hours a day spent with my best friend.

2) My knowledge of cancer and the medical system has improved significantly; I think my previous level of understanding was probably higher than normal due to our unfortunate family history...however, I am now armed with so much information that I can't help but be a strong advocate for prevention as well as a resource for anyone dealing with the process.

3) Increased confidence in myself; conquering simultaneous chemo and radiation treatments (without too much difficultly I might add) will do that for you.

4) I'm more comfortable with my own mortality; luckily, I got to this place early in my journey (it almost seemed like a pre-requisite to moving forward with the process)...although I've accepted dying as a possible outcome, I'm not scared of dying as I'm too busy living.

5) I have a greater appreciation for the subtleties of life; for example, I have always loved nature but my enjoyment and respect for it seems somehow amplified now...the way wind-blown snow clings to the side of a tree or how sunlight hits various objects at different times of the day.

6) Re-connecting with family and friends; we've been in contact with many folks that we haven't seen for many years (isn't it unfortunate how easily people drift apart in our "busy' world)...this interaction has provided immeasurable benefit to my mental state.

7) I discovered my love of writing; my journaling has not only been cathartic and an efficient means of communication, it has also been very enjoyable.

8) I feel closer to my kids; I'm not sure why exactly...perhaps it gets back to the mortality issue somehow and an innate need to teach them as much as possible...to leave my mark before it's too late.

9) I am less guarded, more open; whilst I have not yet progressed to hugging strangers on the street, I do feel that I'm now a warmer, more amiable person.

10) Greater faith in humanity; I fully admit to being a curmudgeon at times in the past, although the current state of the world makes this easy at times... however, the tremendous support we have received from family, close friends and distant acquaintances has reminded me that people aren't that bad after

all...despite our many obvious shortcomings, such as greed and the love of shiny objects, we are social beasts that need each other to survive.

Being A Cancer "Survivor"

In reality, the ugly, not-too-well-known truth about cancer is that it affects you long after its left your body. The physical fatigue, maintenance treatments and weariness is just the tip of the iceberg. The emotional drainage of facing your mortality, sometimes multiple times, the frustration of an all-too-slow recovery and the realization that you may never be your old self again plagues many cancer patients long after their last treatment is over. Not to mention the medical bills...

But finishing treatment is still hailed as a victory, as something that needs to be celebrated, so cancer survivors (and survivors of any tragedy for that matter) become hailed as heroes; physical embodiments of words like "brave."

The thing is, survivors are now expected to act that way - they too often have to put on a happy face because the cancer is "finished". But that expectation is unfair and it's leading to many survivors hiding their true feelings; often not getting help or dealing with it. It's leading to too many feeling ashamed or weak when they don't feel as strong as people think they are.

One website warned that expecting someone to feel glad that they survived cancer is like telling war veterans with PTSD that they should cheer up and just be glad they're alive. It's not always easy being grateful for the worst thing that's ever happened to you.

The Question Of Dying

It's time I brought up the question of spiritual matters. After all, every one of us is going to die sooner or later. We need a worthy response to this most final of all callings. What does life mean, if it only ends in death anyway?

I love Bernie Siegel's masterful aphorism: *death is a form of healing*. For many—and not just cancer sufferers—death brings down a curtain on all our troubles and travail. It is over. No more hurt.

But, as we have seen repeatedly through this text, there is plenty of healing available, if you tackle cancer in the right way—as a psychological issue, as well as a biological one. This is important, because even if you don't get the cure you want, you'll have strength to the end.

It hardly bears repeating that the "quality of life" as you work through this disease is one of the key issues. You can't measure health and life values in terms of days, weeks or months.

To people living with cancer, life is precious. When pain becomes part of each day, of one's daily life, these days are diminished and quality of life is eroded.

The list of damage that pain does to quality of life includes:

- sleep is disturbed
- ability to work is impaired
- exhaustion can become a constant companion
- sadness, depression and worry are commonly felt emotions
- appetite diminishes
- simple pleasures such as enjoying one's family are impaired or given up
- trips and vacations are uncomfortable or impossible
- reluctance to move or exercise is experienced
- feelings of isolation from the world increase
- family and friends who are caregivers become exhausted.

Every cancer patient who has experienced unrelieved pain can provide his or her own list of the damage pain can do to one's life.

Even if you believe that you are psychology strong and can tolerate the pain from cancer or cancer treatments, consider this: by living in pain, you are depriving those who love and care for you the full pleasure of your company. To continue to suffer, especially in light of the fact that very good quality of pain relief is available for almost all cancer pain, is not only hurting yourself, but also those who care for you.

It's important to understand, too, that cancer pain can undermine your ability to fight your cancer. If pain has you in its grip, your appetite diminishes. This means you may not be receiving sufficient nutrition to retain energy which, in turn, leads to exhaustion and feelings of sadness and depression. As this cycle continues, a person is worn down gradually, may become more vulnerable to infection, and the ability to withstand necessary cancer treatments may diminish.

So positive psychology, of the kind I have been writing about at length in this book, is absolutely crucial.

SHUN NEGATIVE WORDS AND PHRASES

"Sticks and stones may break my bones but words will never hurt me." We all know this simple roundelay. But it's not true. Words are very powerful and used wrongly can most definitely hurt you, even kill you.

The truth is, as Wendell Johnson tells us in his book *Your Most Enchanted Listener* (Harper and Bros: New York 1956), words have a tremendous impact on the speaker. Far more than the recipient they are aimed at. This is a little-known but crucial point of psychology.

It's not just a question of "I can, I can, I can," as the little engine said. Or "I can't, I can't, I can't." If a man speaks to a woman and yells "You lousy bitch," he is hurting himself as well as the woman. To speak ill is to think ill and to think ill is poison to the mind.

Yet slovenly and destructive talk is very commonplace. I am not here to moralize about eff*ing and blinding as we say in England, or cussin' and swearin' as Americans say.

The really important message is that, if you speak bad things about your life, you will have a negative impact on your heart, mind and physiology. I don't even care if you believe that at this stage; just pay attention.

I had a woman once with cancer who spoke vilely to her husband. The marriage was all but done; and she kept yelling at him, "You make me sick." So the prophecy came true and she obligingly got sick. Almost to the point of death.

I coached her to listen to what she was *actually* saying... she thought she was abusing her husband, but follow the words carefully: she was wishing sickness on herself.

Yes wishing. So she got cancer.

This is something hard to teach but a brilliant insight: to speak a state or condition is to "wish" it. "I'm broke" is a wish. So is, "I'm going to make it on Broadway."

"I have a stage IV cancer," is a wish. Read again on page 40 what I said about denials: patients who confidently said, "I don't have cancer, this is just a temporary state of affairs" might have seemed foolish dreamers. But for many, it was just a wish... and it came true. That's how powerful words can be.

Writers are fond of quoting Masaru Emoto and his work supposedly showing that bad words will spoil water crystals (ice) but good words will make water form beautiful shapes and patterns. Unfortunately (for me), Emoto discredited himself. He admitted to picking only the best results, that made his point. You can't do that in science; it's called dishonesty! You have to take whatever comes.

As my friend Stanford University Professor Emeritus William Tiller points out, it is extremely easy to manipulate the crystalline structure of water, especially by adding contaminants or tinkering with the cooling rate of the water. In Dr. Tiller's words, "In Dr. Emoto's experiments, [supercooling] was neither controlled nor measured, a necessary requirement to be fulfilled if one wanted to prove that it was the new factor of specific human intention that was causative."[Tiller, William A. "What the BLEEP Do We Know!?: A Personal Perspective." *Vision in Action*, Volume Two, 2004. Pg. 18. http://www.via-visioninaction.org/via-li/journals/What_the_Bleep_Perspectives_Vol2_No3-4.pdf]

Apparently, Emoto's experimental protocols are so lacking as to be unrepeatable, and even the most basic attempts at scientific controls are absent.

But that aside, it does not prove that words and thoughts cannot affect physical structure. They can. I just don't quote Emoto any more and remain dispassionate.

More valuable evidence comes from anecdotal sources. If you search YouTube long enough (the evil goons at Google are trying increasingly to hide anything they say whiffs of a miracle cure—the determination is made by some half-assed teen who knows nothing about medicine and healing), you will find a filmed instance of a 3-inch diameter bladder cancer being chanted and wished away in just a matter of minutes!

The healing took place at a medicine-less hospital in Beijing, China. This was achieved by what presenter Gregg Braden describes as a lost modality of prayer. Three health workers stood by the woman, working with the energy in the patient's body and the feelings in their bodies, and chanted a word they had agreed reinforced the feeling that the patient is already healed.

The ultrasound video camera shows the tumor shrinking literally before our eyes until, after only a few minutes, it is gone.

Notice they were perceiving the woman as *fully healed*. They were not chanting "Bad cancer, you must go away..." which, of course, would wish the cancer into place.

This is why we must all be careful with wishes and affirmations; that we do not inadvertently reinforce the negative by putting it in place, in order to wish it away!

Does all this seem a bit much? I'm not suggesting you rush off to Beijing and find these three practitioners. But I am urging you to understand the power of the words in your mouth and what you say about yourself and your state of health.

SINGING AWAY CANCER?

Here's a little more background to the possible powers of chanting.

If you are not familiar with the work of Fabien Maman, it's time you were. He was able to destroy cancer cells by singing at them. No, really! Music, after all, is a psychological phenomenon, as well as a resonance effect!

Maman is a French composer and bio-energeticist, who explored and documented the influence of sound waves on the cells of the body. He was fascinated with energetic healing techniques, and wondered if we are really affected biologically, or even changed by music? If so, how deeply does sound travel into our bodies?

He began a year-and-a-half study joined by Helene Grimal, an ex-nun who had left the convent to become a drummer. She supported herself musically in her profession as a biologist at the French National Center for Scientific Research in Paris. Together they studied the effect of low volume sound (30-40 decibels) on human cells.

The pair mounted a camera on a microscope where they had placed slides of human uterine cancer cells. They proceeded to play various acoustic instruments (guitar, gong, xylophone as well as voice) for periods of twenty-minute duration, while they observed the effect on the cells.

Sounding the notes of the Ionian Scale (nine musical notes C-D-E-F-G-A-B and C and D from the next octave above), the cellular structures quickly disorganized. Fourteen minutes was enough time to explode the cell when he used these nine different frequencies, reported Maman.

The most dramatic influence on the cells came from the human voice: when he *sang* the same scale, the cancer cells literally "exploded" in less than 10 minutes.

The vibration of sound literally transforms the cell structure. As the voice intensifies and time passes with no break in sound, the vibratory rate becomes too powerful, and the cells cannot adapt or stabilize themselves. Therefore, the cell dies because it is not able to accommodate its structure and synchronize with the collection of sound. Cells cannot live in an atmosphere of dissonance and they cannot become resonant with the body. Therefore, the tumor cells destabilize, disorganize, disintegrate, explode and are ultimately destroyed in the presence of pure sound.

What was especially exciting to me was that one particular note—A at 440 Hertz—seemed to carry the most healing power. Maman has produced numerous photographic images, showing that A (the note an orchestra tunes to) turned cell energy fields Indian pink. Pink is a healing color and associated with love, as we all know. This Indian pink effect on cells appears, no matter what instrument the note A is sounded on.

As Maman said excitedly: What if, for 20 minutes, radio stations and hospital intercoms played pieces in the key of A? What if children sang songs, mothers hummed to their babies and public PA systems all broadcast this note? Perhaps for 20 minutes, at least, our world could be harmonized.

What if, indeed?

A full treatment of healing by musical resonance is not appropriate here but if you are indeed interested, then you can follow up with Maman's book *The Role of Music in the Twenty-First Century* (Redondo Beach, CA, 1997). You will also enjoy *The Healing Forces of Music* by Randall McClellan (Element, Rockport MA, 1991).

WHERE IS GOD IN ALL THIS?

There's a decades-old story that goes around. Bernie Siegel tells a version of it in his book *Love, Medicine and Miracles*. I'll re-tell it in my own words, the way I would over a glass of wine beside the Adriatic...

It concerns a man who had terminal cancer. He wasn't doing well. But he remained optimistic and told everybody, "I'll be OK. God is with me and I'll be healed."

He held to this, even when a nutritionist tried to intervene and show him how he could at least slow down the tumor growth. "I'll be just fine," he told the nutritionist. "God will save me, I know."

A new oncologist tried to get some sense into the man and talked to him of exciting new possibilities. "I don't need an oncologist," he responded. "I have God and I know God will save me."

He was so stubborn, they tried with a psychologist but he got nowhere either. "It's not about my state of mind," said the man. "I'm just confident that God will save me."

So the man died.

When he got to Heaven, he was plenty mad, and demanded why God had not saved him, when he had such implicit faith in the Lord?

I sent you a nutritionist, an oncologist and a psychologist," boomed the Big Voice. "You refused them all. So I could not help you."

This is not just a cruel joke. It makes an important point, which is that God is not going to do your thinking for you. In fact God seems a little indifferent on the whole. We were given the power of thinking and reason and I believe that basically we are supposed to get on with it.

I know that won't suit everyone. There are people who loudly sing God's praises when they have a lucky break: "The Good Lord saved me from cancer," such a person will whisper reverently. But when I child gets run over on the railway tracks and horribly crushed, that wasn't God, apparently.

Well, why not?

I think God is often used as an excuse to deny responsibility in life, when the exact opposite is required of us.

Forgiveness Is Godliness

Now I have a couple of suggestions. Firstly, what we may think of as God has another name: love. Love is something that none of us can do without. Love interweaves with all the threads and layers of our lives. How we deliver ourselves up to love is something that God, if there is such a One, expects us to get right.

Life is too short for petty bickering, miserable whining and bitter accusations. Even if people do seem to do bad things to you, you have one overarching choice: to forgive. You can release yourself from suffering at the hands of others, if you learn to forgive.

There is a big misunderstanding about forgiveness, which prevents people being more loving, understanding and forgiving, and that is the belief or the fixed idea that to forgive someone is somehow to "let the person off"; to excuse him or her. Whereas he or she should be made to feel bad, to take the blame that is rightly theirs, to suffer, maybe, and realize that what they did to you was wrong.

There are several things wrong with this all-too-common idea. To begin with, people very rarely admit or even recognize that they have done something wrong. When it comes down to it—if matters were thrown open to public opinion—very often outsiders wouldn't see any big deal either. They might wonder why you are making such a fuss!

Be humble and let go of the feeling you are entitled to justice.

The truth is, it is a pointless and unrewarding task to try to make someone feel they have done wrong when they don't themselves see it. You are not going to change that. So why set yourself up for misery?

Secondly, there is the mistaken belief that when the person who hurt you admits they were in the wrong, you will start to feel better, to be healed. But it's nonsense! The ONLY thing that can change how you feel is you! You create your feelings... all of them, not someone else.

To say to a person "You hurt me," is silly and totally untrue. You hurt yourself. You turn on your feelings, no-one else does that! Being hurt is a choice. Choose again, I say. Choose freedom instead.

But the third, and biggest, mistake is to fail to see that forgiveness is something you do that will release your own suffering. It has nothing to do with the person you believe hurt you, nothing at all.

To forgive someone for a wrong they did, even just an imagined wrong, is to be kind and gentle with *yourself*. Forgiveness releases you, the sufferer. This really is true and if you have not tried it, you may be unsure. But the moment you start forgiving others, you will see an amazing transformation in yourself.

Your pain will lessen. You will feel warmer, more centered and more loving.

Remember: forgiveness is an act of loving yourself. It is really unimportant what effect it has on the person who hurt you.

But often, you may be surprised, what good it does and how it can change other people's feelings, as well as your own!

There is a lovely Hawaiian practice of full reconciliation, healing and forgiveness called *ho'oponopono*. You should try to make it a habit. In Hawai'i the ritual involved an elder, a kahuna or wise person, and all the family. Everyone has to spill their guts and get it all off their chests. No-one is allowed to leave the room till all the skeletons, resentments, guilt and other ugly feelings are expressed. Only when there has been full clearing and resolution is the ritual ended.

But it can be done alone or in small groups or pairs. If you are on your own, this is how I teach *ho'oponopono*:

Now...

One at a time, say (out loud) the following heartfelt statements. Truly... mean what you say.

To yourself say: *"I'm sorry. Please forgive me. Thank you. I love you."*

To your nearest and dearest on Earth say: *"I'm sorry. Please forgive me. Thank you. I love you."*

To the Earth herself say: *"I'm sorry. Please forgive me. Thank you. I love you."*

To God say: *"I'm sorry. Please forgive me. Thank you. I love you."*

Having activated and opened your heart chakra... you should find it easier to forgive.

Think of a person who has hurt you and say the following; really mean it:

I fully and freely forgive you. The past is gone. All wounds are healed. I wish you well in life. May you have peace and blessings. May you find love.

Now think of someone else you feel has hurt you. Say to them also—and really mean it...

I fully and freely forgive you. The past is gone. All wounds are healed. I wish you well in life. May you have peace and blessings. May you find love.

Think of times in your own life when your wrong actions have hurt or disappointed others. None of us is perfect. None of us is without fault. It is much easier to forgive others, when we bear in mind our own weaknesses and failings.

Find another person you feel has hurt you. Say to them also—and really mean it...

I fully and freely forgive you. The past is gone. All wounds are healed. I wish you well in life. May you have peace and blessings. May you find love.

Wherever you are stuck and upset with someone you feel has hurt you unjustifiably, love *yourself* enough to forgive that person and so find your own release and freedom from suffering.

Say to each person you think of, say:

I fully and freely forgive you. The past is gone. All wounds are healed. I wish you well in life. May you have peace and blessings. May you find love.

You can repeat this process often. You don't need to dream up new offenders each time. Just be sure to conjure up the feeling of full and loving forgiveness.

I wish you all-healing.

[Note: it might be best not to tell the person you are forgiving him or her. That can come over as a little arrogant and supercilious even. Forgiveness works without telling anyone at all]

GOD AS A STATE OF GRACE

The other suggestion, or role model, if you like, is God as a state of grace or a state of being. I can't hack the idea of God as a hairy old fart in the sky, who hates women, has anger management issues and eavesdrops your thoughts to see if you are wicked, with a view to torturing you through all eternity. I mean... c'mon!

It doesn't make sense.

George Carlin is particularly funny in this respect. He says: "...tell the people that the paint is wet and they will want to touch it, just to be sure. But tell them an invisible man in the sky created all things, and they will believe you!"

But what if God is not a quasi-creature but is a state of being; a feeling of awesome, unconditional love; a condition of wonderful connectedness and peace, that makes you feel exquisite joy, almost to the point of hurting?

Many mystics have described a connection with God in those terms (well, a little more flowery but you get the point). Teresa d' Avila, for example, was renowned for her ecstatic feelings when she connected with God, a moment of which was captured by a lovely statue of her created by Gian Lorenzo Bernini and now rests in the Santa Maria della Vittoria in Rome.

The point, surely, is that if God is depicted as some almighty figure or form, He becomes inaccessible. If it is a state of being, we can all aspire to it, in the end.

I'm thinking now especially of the story of Anita Moorjani, which should be an inspiration to all cancer sufferers. Her story went viral very quickly. She tells it so well...

Anita had end-stage cancer (Hodgkin's Lymphoma), and was being cared for at home. She was connected to an oxygen tank, and had a full time nurse. But on this morning, February 2nd 2006, she did not wake up.

"I had fallen into a coma. My husband called the doctor who said I needed to be rushed to hospital. The senior oncologist looked at me and told my husband that it was now the end, and that my organs were shutting down. I would probably not make it beyond the next 36 hours..."

This is about as bad as it gets, surely?

"I thought that I was drifting in and out of consciousness during this time, because I was aware of everything that was going on around me. But it was confirmed to me later by my family and the doctors that I was in a coma the whole time. I saw and heard the conversations between my husband and the doctors taking place outside my room, about 40 feet away down a hallway. I was later able to verify this conversation to my shocked husband. Then I actually "crossed over" to another dimension, where I was engulfed in a total feeling of love. I also experienced extreme clarity of why I had the cancer, why I had come into this life in the first place, what role everyone in my family played in my life in the grand scheme of things, and generally how life works. The clarity and understanding I obtained in this state is almost indescribable. Words seem to limit the experience — I was at a place where I understood how much more there is than what we are able to conceive in our 3-dimensional world. I realized what a gift life was, and that I was sur-rounded by loving spiritual beings, who were always around me, even when I did not know it..."

It was at this moment, Anita tells us, that she came to realize that God was not a being but a state; a state of infinite, unconditional love.

"At first, I did not want to come back, because my body was very sick, and I did not want to come back into this body as the organs had already stopped functioning and I had all these open skin lesions. But it seemed that, almost immediately, I became aware that if I chose life, my body would heal very quickly. I would see a difference in not months or weeks, but days!

And that's exactly what happened. From having lesions the size of lemons from the base of her skull to her lower abdomen, within days all the tumors were gone. In less than a week doctors could find nothing to take a biopsy from. They put it down to her suddenly responding to the chemo. Because the doctors were unable to explain what was going on, they subjected Ani-ta to test after test, all of which turned out normal. Even a full body scan showed her tissues were back to normal. The doctors were so confused, they even made the radiologist repeat the scan.

"After what I have seen," Anita says, "I realize that absolutely anything is possible, and that we did not come here to suffer. Life is supposed to be great, and we are very, very loved."

I hope with that comforting note, that all my readers, both patients and loved ones, will realize that cancer has the power to heal, as well as the power to kill.

In fact one of the sayings I have lately adopted is that cancer is a teaching disease. It will teach us more about life and death than any books, films or scriptures!

Let's leave it at that.

CANCER IS LOVE AT THE WRONG LEVEL

Thorwald Dethlefsen, in his delightful book The Healing Power Of Disease, makes an interesting political association between cancer and human behavior. It's about wholeness and the body politic. The inventor of the term holism, remember, was a statesman: South African military leader, Jan Smuts.

Every whole that we perceive is part of a greater whole and is also an assembly of many lesser wholes. So, for example, a wood is not only part of a greater whole, the countryside, but is composed of many lesser wholes—the individual trees growing in it.

In the same way each human being is part of the greater whole of humanity. But we ourselves also consist of a collection of organs, which are smaller wholes; and each organ, in turn, is made up of a multiplicity of cells which are even smaller wholes. We could theoretically continue to extend this hierarchy in either direction.

The core concept of holism, as first expressed by Jan Smuts, is that the whole is not just the sum of its parts. The whole is something new, something extra, something that doesn't exist when you remove any of the parts. Biologically, in health, each part of a complex organism functions in such a way that each part works towards the success of the whole. So our organs for example work towards our survival as a living creature.

Each whole system can cope with the failure of a few of its constituent parts without much damage, but there is a limit. Beyond that limit, the whole begins to break up!

So it is in politics: a state or country can cope with some of its citizens refusing to work, behaving anti-socially or becoming rebel activists, working against the government. However if the number of dissenters grows too large, the whole is threatened and the government tries to prevent that, by removing dissenters from the pool, before it is overthrown.

This is a broader principle: if there are too few elements working for the good of the whole, or too many working against it, then the whole may perish.

Dethlefsen likens our own bodies to a state or country and cancer cells he sees as a rebellious element, which wants to follow its own path, regardless of the consequences to the whole. A cancer, as I have often remarked, is not some alien object dropped into the body from a flying saucer, but a part of the body politic that is turned to a different path. In other words, cancer cells were once normal citizens but have turned bad.

The cancer seems not to care if the host dies. But this is faulty logic: if the host dies, the cancer too will die. In other words, cancer cells have become reckless and shortsighted. The cancer too is on a path to demise, along with the host.

But, as Dethlefsen remarks, isn't this also true also of human behavior at this time? Mankind is trying to assure its own survival on the same basis as cancerous tissue, which is to grab everything needed or desired, and ignore the consequences further down the line. We humans have become a kind of cancer to our planet!

In that sense, Dethlefsen points out, cancer is more or less a projection of our era and our collective outlook on the planet. What we undergo inwardly as cancer is merely what we ourselves are doing outwardly to our own environment.

> "Our whole rationale is just like that of the cancer cell. So rapid and successful is our expansion that we too can barely cope with our supply problems. Our communications systems extend worldwide, yet still we cannot communicate with our neighbors or partners. We have leisure, yet we do not know what to do with it. We produce and destroy foodstuffs, purely in order to manipulate prices. We can travel

the whole world and still do not know ourselves. Our current philoso-phy knows no other goal but growth and progress."

Isn't that exactly like a cancer behaves? The cancer-cell simply cannot hold a candle to the blindness and short-sightedness of contemporary humanity.

His rant continues, "For the sake of pursuing economic expansion, we have for decades been exploiting our environment as both larder and host, only to be astonished by the sudden realization that the death of the host also involves the death of humanity itself. We regard the whole world is a quarry to be mined — whether for plants, animals or raw materials. The one and only reason why it is all there, it seems, is so that we can spread ourselves across the face of the earth *ad infinitum.*

"In the light of this behavior, how can we possibly have the gall or sheer, bare-faced cheek to complain about cancer?"

There's more: "It's not a question of conquering cancer: it is merely a ques-tion of understanding it, so that we can then learn to understand ourselves too. How keen we are to smash the mirror whenever we do not like the look of our face! If we become cancerous, it is because we are cancerous."

Phew, heavy stuff!

Dialogue With Cancer

Something I do with all Supernoetics® piloting clients is to get him or her dialoguing with the cancer: What does it want to tell you? What do you want to say to it? Backwards and forwards, question and answer.

Cancer gives us an opportunity to discover the extent of our own misunder-standings and false reasoning.

For some of you that may sound strange but for most of you, I don't think so. You'll get it!

The point is, cancer is telling your something, even if it's only that your health is in ruins. But it's more subtle than that. Cancer-cells are rogues that have gone off the rails and turned bandit. We need to know why and what to do about it.

Healing then is a matter of re-uniting, of regaining one-ness, restoring that holism. You cannot be whole in health while part of your biological creature is attacking the rest of your tissues.

It comes down to love. Remember the technique of the late Dr. Patrick Kingsley I wrote up for you on page 72. Love those cancer cells and they might just come back into the fold, give up the rebellion and start a healing process.

While ever the cancer cell believes in a separate world to "self", then conflict ensues. But once it is understood that we are a part of the greater whole, the cancer too will yield. That's why so many holistic and gentle cures are effective against this fearful disease. Gentle is loving! Inviting! To seek to kill and destroy the cancer is to alienate it, to reinforce its whole doctrine of Me-and-You.

This doctrine is fatal.

And the only remedy is love, says Dethlefsen. "Love heals, because it opens up the barriers and lets in the other with a view to becoming one with it. Those who are in love do not put their ego first, but experience a greater wholeness: they feel as though they themselves were their lovers."

Nor does this only happen in the human context. It seems to apply in our attitude to animals too.

In fact, Dethlefsen goes as far as to remark that *cancer is a sign of unexpressed love—indeed, it is a perverted form of love.*

"Love transcends all bounds and barriers. In love, the opposites unite and fuse together. Love is union with all; it extends to everything and shrinks at nothing. Love has no fear even of death—for love is life. Those who fail consciously to live out this love run the risk that their love will descend into the body, where it will seek to realise its inner laws in the form of cancer.

"Cancer cells, too, transcend all bounds and barriers: cancer, after all, dissolves the various organs' individualities.

"Cancer, too, extends to everything and shrinks at nothing (metastasis).

"Cancer cells, too, have no fear of death."

"Cancer is love at the wrong level," says Dethlefsen. "Total union is something that can be realised only at the level of total consciousness, not within matter, for matter is consciousness's shadow."

[quotes from Dethlefsen T., *The Healing Power Of Illness*, Sentient Publications, Boulder, CO, 2016, pp. 241-250. Co-author Reudiger Dahlke MD. Translated by Peter Lemesurier]

Powerful and moving stuff, to suppose then that cancer is the symptom of misunderstood love. Cancer treats true love only with respect. The symbol of true love is the heart. Interestingly the heart is the only organ that cannot be attacked by cancer!

Go figure.

Let me finish with my favorite quote about the power of love. It's from preacher Emmet Fox, in his book Sermon On The Mount:

> "There is no difficulty that enough love will not conquer;
> No disease that enough love will not heal;
> No door that enough love will not open;
> No gulf that enough love will not bridge;
> No wall that enough love will not throw down;
> No sin that enough love will not redeem....
> It makes no difference how deeply seated may be the trouble;
> How hopeless the outlook;
> How muddled the tangle;
> How great the mistake....
> A sufficient realization of love will dissolve it all"

What more is there to say?

PART 4

DOES PRAYER HELP? YOU BET!

And I don't just mean praying because you are facing death—I mean prayer as a healing tool!

In Part 2 I talked about the incredibly powerful influence of mind over health and how negative emotions MUST be addressed, in order to survive cancer— otherwise it will probably come back!

Going further than that we can look at the spiritual dimension of healing.

We can call on God, or simply look to Higher Self, or both. There are people who call for guides and angels to help them in the healing process. This is all valid stuff at the individual level.

Prayer, or course, is part of this dimension. Many people have been willing to testify that prayer alone and God's intervention is what saved them.

In medicine, we see the touch of spirit all the time in cases of "spontaneous remission." If it happens at a prayer meeting, then God gets the credit, other- wise it is just one of those inexplicable marvels of the human body.

Dr. Randolph Byrd, a Christian cardiologist, conducted a study in 1984 that has led to a resurgence of scientific evaluation of the effect of prayer on healing.

393 patients, admitted to the coronary care unit at San Francisco General Hospital, over a 10 month period were randomly selected, by computer, to either a 201 patient control group or the 192 patients who were prayed for daily by 5-7 people in home prayer groups. This was a randomized, dou-

ble-blind experiment in which neither the patients, nurses, nor doctors knew which group the patients were in.

Dr. Byrd discovered a definite pattern of obvious differences between the control group and those prayed for:

None of those prayed for required endotracheal intubation compared with twelve in the control group requiring the insertion of an artificial airway in the throat.

The prayed for group experienced fewer cases of pneumonia and cardio-pulmonary arrests. Those prayed for were five times less likely to require antibiotics.

The prayed for group were three times less likely to develop pulmonary edema, a condition where the lungs fill with fluid.

Fewer patients in the prayed for group died.

Dr. Larry Dossey, M.D. states, referring to Dr. Byrd's experiment, that "If the technique being studied had been a new drug or a surgical procedure instead of prayer, it would almost certainly have been heralded as some sort of breakthrough"

The importance of this experiment is that it stands up to scientific scrutiny. Dr. William Nolan, who has written a book debunking faith healing, acknowledged, " It sounds like this study will stand up to scrutiny…maybe we doctors ought to be writing on our order sheets, 'pray 3 times a day.' If it works, it works."

Extensive experimental evidence for "spiritual healing" is one of the best kept secrets in medical science.

Daniel J. Benor, M.D., an American psychiatrist working in England, surveyed all such healing studies published in the English language prior to 1990. His search turned up 131 studies, most of them on non-humans. In 56 of these studies, there was less than one chance in a hundred that the positive results were due to chance. In an additional 21 studies, the possibility of a chance explanation was between 2 and 5 chances in a 100. A complete list of Dr. Benor's compilation is available as *Spiritual Healing: Professional Supplement (Healing Research)*, Vision Publications, Southfield, MI, 2002.

As an example of his compilation, 60 subjects not known to have healing ability were able to both impede and stimulate significantly the growth of cultures of bacteria.

In another experiment, volunteers were asked to alter the genetic ability of a strain of bacteria to metabolize the sugar lactose. The results indicated that the bacteria indeed mutated in the direction desired by the subjects.

Medical journals, until recently, have generally refused to publish studies on healing.

In December of 1998 issue of JAMA the *Journal of the American Medical Association*, journalist Mike Mitka commented on the number of research articles available to physicians wanting to incorporate spirituality into their treatment arsenal [JAMA (1998) 280:1896–7]. JAMA specifically referred to the following works:

Duke University reports that people who attended religious services at least once a week and prayed or studied the Bible at least daily had consistently lower blood pressure than those who did so less frequently or not at all.

The Journal of the National Cancer Institute reported that studies indicate many cancer patients, in particular, rely on religion and spirituality after their diagnosis.

A University of Michigan study involving 93 of 106 women under treatment for various stages of uterine and ovarian cancer, said their religious lives helped them sustain hope.

Edward Creagan, M.D., of the Division of Medical Oncology at the Mayo Clinic, said that "among the coping methods of long-term cancer survivors, the predominant strategy is spiritual." Creagan complains that psychosocial interventions can be life enhancing in sharp contrast to the guilt-ridden programs of some alternative practitioners, a point worth bearing in mind (see my remarks on page 58). A social support system and an element of spirituality and religion seem to be the most consistent predictors of quality of life and possible survival among patients with advanced malignant disease, he says. [Attitude and disposition: do they make a difference in cancer survival? Mayo Clin Proc. 1997 Feb;72(2):160-4].

In 1996, Time magazine did a cover story on the belief in the power of prayer for health and healing. The poll found that 82 percent of the adult Americans believed in the healing power of personal prayer, 73 percent believed praying for someone can help cure their illness, and 64 percent believed doctors should pray with patients if requested to.

Newsweek confirmed the findings, a year later with its own poll, in which 79 percent of respondents who said they prayed regularly declared that they believe God answers prayers for healing.

The Lancet, a British medical publication, reported: "Of 296 physicians surveyed during the October, 1996, meeting of the American Academy of Family Physicians, 99% were convinced that religious beliefs can heal, and 75% believed that prayers of others could promote a patient's recovery. [The Lancet: Volume 353, No. 9153, p664–667, 20 February 1999]

Yet skeptics continue to trash the concept of prayer healing. One commentator (www.wired.com) asked the question "Is This Even Theoretically Possible?" How vacuously unscientific an approach to enquiry is that?

Sceptics lean heavily on a recent (2006) large medical study by Benson, Dusek, et. al., which supposedly found that long distance intercessory prayers, offered by strangers, had no effect on the recovery of people who were undergoing heart surgery. The study begun almost a decade ago involved more than 1,800 patients in six hospitals at a cost of $2.4 million. By the current scientific model this study was "rigorously designed", it was said.

In fact it was a sham. The people who prayed were inexperienced and used an absurd "intellectualized" technique that no intercessory healer would dream of doing. The participants were given only the patients' first names and the first initials of their last names. This is probably not a serious obstacle to an experienced healer but for an inexperienced person it might nullify their ability to connect and provide healing. Participants were instructed to include the phrase "for a successful surgery with a quick, healthy recovery and no complications."

It could never work done Benson's way. And I wouldn't be surprised if he planned it that way. Researchers do.

[Benson, Herbert, Dusek, Jeffery A., et. al., "Study of the Therapeutic Effects of Intercessory Prayer (STEP) in Cardiac Bypass Patients: A Multicenter Randomized Trial of Uncertainty and Certainty of Receiving Intercessory Prayer," American Heart Journal, Vol. 151, No. 4, April 2006, pp. 934-942].

A better double-blind randomized study of distant healing on a population with advanced AIDS was carried out by Fred Sicher, Elisabeth Targ, et. al.

Unlike the Benson study, the Sicher/Targ study selected experienced healers from various backgrounds who chose their own techniques. The ability to sharply focus one's intention to affect a person at a distant location is a skill that these individuals spent a lifetime developing.

Each healer received a packet that included a 5x7-inch color photograph of the target individual. In subtle energy healing practices a full name, photograph, or DNA sample (like a strand of hair) normally serves as an "address" for non-local distant healing.

In contrast to relying on a word phrase, experienced healers usually focus upon a feeling state of love and connect to the heart of the target person.

The Sicher/Targ study concluded that there were positive therapeutic effects of distant healing. The results showed "decreased medical utilization, fewer and less severe new illnesses, and improved mood for the treated group compared with the controls."

[F. Sicher, E. Targ, D. Moore, and HS Smith. A Randomized Double-Blind Study of the Effect of Distant Healing in a Population with Advanced AIDS - Report of a Small Scale Study; Western Journal of Medicine; December 1998; 169:356-363]

HERE'S WHAT I KNOW

All this emphasis on whether or not distant intercessory prayer works is irrelevant and rather distracting. To me what matters in prayer is that the individual focuses intently on communication with his or her God or Higher Power. The very intensity of prayer has an effect on the one who prays that is vivid and real and is equivalent to direct intervention from above.

No-one can want something for us (like a healing) more than we want it for ourselves. So *personal prayer* is the issue. For that there can be no double-blind trials. I regard it as conceited and impertinent that scientists should presume to try and "test" prayer in any such way.

Prayer is unique and personal and neither requires testing or proof, nor is it susceptible to any kind of validation, in my view.

Those who pray can and should believe whatever they want. It doesn't even matter whether the desired change comes from within or from above. It happens. And who could possibly prove it was not from God or Higher Power but just a psychological adaptation?

Some truths are simply not separable from the remainder of reality.

Dr Winston Morrow MD tells a good story which, although not directly about cancer healing, will give the reader a vivid illustration of how powerful prayer healing can be:

> Since 1988, when God miraculously healed me from having to have my left arm amputated at the shoulder, I have prayed for all of my patients.
>
> I have seen new shoulders, confirmed by before and after X-rays, tumors the size of grapefruits disappear and so very many obvious spontaneous and instantaneous healings that I can only conclude that God supernaturally intervened.
>
> In the case of my healing, I had a white count of 75,000, my arm was swollen to almost twice the size of my other arm, it was blue and green with obvious gangrene, and the pain was so intense that I could not bear it.
>
> After I was told, "we have to amputate your arm at the shoulder to-morrow morning, because the IV antibiotics are not working and your whole body is infected and your heart will literally turn to mush", I checked out of the hospital.
>
> A patient of mine told me that God would not let that happen, almost had to drag me into my own office, and began to pray and I was be-ginning to get upset at her audacity, almost to the point of anger... Suddenly, I felt 10,000 degrees of sweet heat start at the top of my head and fill my body...instantly, not 5 minutes or an hour, but in-stantly I got a new arm, no swelling, no discoloration, no pain...
>
> This event was the impetus for my praying for all of my patients be-fore treatment begins. I do it with them, asking God for wisdom, and asking his Holy Spirit to do those things that I cannot do as a man. Sometimes the anointing is so strong that it is obvious that the Spirit of God is present.

I thank Him constantly for hitting me over the head and waking up this Christian who didn't believe that God is in the healing business today. I thought that it all stopped with the apostles.

BEYOND PRAYER

One of the greatest healers in the world, a modest, unassuming man, who makes no claims that God has chosen him specially, is Matthew Manning. He lectures and demonstrates his techniques all over the world. He has been involved in more scientific research and testing than any other healer in the world and has addressed the Royal Society of Medicine and spoken to MPs in the Houses of Parliament about his healing work.

[http://www.matthewmanning.com]

Here's a typical healing story:

Ricky visited Matthew after a biopsy confirmed cancer of the vocal chords. He then underwent a second biopsy for the surgical "stripping" of the site of the cancer. His consultant told him that radiotherapy would be needed if there were signs of further invasion after his throat had settled down from the biopsy.

After a healing session with Matthew Ricky wrote with typical British humor, "When I saw you, I told you that I felt something happening in my throat during the session and that when I concentrated something in my head seemed to be 'in tune'. Once I was in the car, I tried my voice – amazing! Pavarotti won't have sleepless nights yet, but what a difference! When I got home I tried it out on the family and they were speechless, which makes a change for them. Now I can order a pint in a pub without being ignored."

Ricky returned to hospital for a check-up after his second healing session with Matthew. His throat specialist described as "quite remarkable" the speed and degree of healing that had taken place in his throat. He had several further healing sessions "just in case the Phantom of the Opera croaks and gets stuck in the chandelier", and was eventually discharged by the hospital.

Synchronicity Rocks!

I found an interesting synchronicity in starting correspondence with Matthew. In his book *One Foot In The Stars,* he describes a seminal moment in his spiritual development, which was an experiment following Konstantin Raudive's book on electronic voice phenomena (EVP).

Well, Raudive's name isn't exactly on everyone's lips. But I had already written about him myself, in my book Virtual Medicine. Raudive was an Latvian researcher, investigating the amazing phenomenon of voices from people who were (definitely) dead being picked up on electromagnetic recording devices (in those days it was magnetic reel-to-reel wire recorders, followed later by tape).

In Virtual Medicine, I have introduced a whole new chapter about this, and similar phenomena, that I titled "Biology Beyond The Grave" (echoing an earlier chapter, written in 1999, which I had titled "Biology Beyond The Skin"). My take on it was that the field effect survives death. Advanced physics not only says that we may live on after death but the we MUST, by the nature of physics, survive as an energy and information field. Perhaps that's all there is to "ghosts"!

Matthew describes how he and several school friends got hold of a tape recorder and tried to make contact with the "other side". After carefully checking the tape was blank and several failed attempts, one of the boys suggested summoning Hitler and inviting him to speak.

Well, the Fuehrer declined apparently. But when played back, this "blank tape" now contained the crunch of hundreds of marching footsteps, brass bands and a very military impression, which eventually broke into gunfire and running feet.

[Incidentally, for those of the faithful who may be troubled, don't be concerned. Even the Vatican accepts this phenomenon of EVP and more than one priest has been involved in making recordings, including the President of the Papal Academy. His Holiness the Pope, no less, pronounced on EVP and said that it was a good thing, because it helped the faithful to be assured there really was life after death.]

I'm sorry for this diversion but I thought you would find it interesting and you need to read it along with section #47 Death Is Not The End

So back to spiritual healing and using Matthew Manning as a fine example of what is possible. It is interesting to report on a remarkable research trial, carried out at the Science Unlimited Research Foundation in San Antonio, Texas, under Dr. John Kmetz. The test was to see if Matthew could influence cancer cells, held in a flask in his hand, but otherwise untouched.

The cells in question were from a famous line of "immortal" cancer cells called the He-La strain (they were taken from a black American woman called Henrietta Lafayette, who died of cancer on October 4, 1951).

Manning describes how he held the flask in his hand and visualized the cancer cells surrounded in white light, and spoke (silently) to the cells, suggesting that their purpose on this level of reality had ended and they had to go elsewhere. He repeated this on 30 successive flasks, sometimes trying to influence them from a distance, without even touching the flasks.

As a control, another person who was not a spiritual healer was asked to hold similar flasks and mimic Manning's every movement. Yet another set of controls were kept in a remote part of the building, untouched by experimenters until the counting began.

The results were irrefutable: in 27 out the 30 test flasks that Manning actually "healed", there were drops in the cancer cell count, varying in degree from 200- 1,000%. None of the control flasks—either the ones handled or the ones in a remote part of the building—showed any significant changes whatever.

In 1986 Manning was asked to address orthodox doctors about cancer at the Royal Society of Medicine (of which I am a member, though it is much diminished of late and no longer requires election to membership). I wasn't there that night but he put his case well I'm sure, despite the audience sitting quietly grinding their teeth.

I like Manning, by the way, because he's modest and includes his notable failures in his book, not just the spectacular success. In fact that leads quite neatly to my final conclusion, which is this: spiritual healing clearly works and has a place. But it seems very unpredictable; there is no way to know in advance who will benefit and who won't. That means there must be many disappointments. But spiritual healing is no less valid for that.

I do not propose to dress all this up with quotations from quantum physics, as is the fashion. To me there will always be something "beyond physics". If you are suffering from any pain, any disease, I hope you will be able to contact help from this other realm and be benefited it, with or without a healer's help.

I suppose spiritual healing leads naturally towards this final topic...

DEATH IS NOT THE END

It may seem strange to conclude a book on cancer cures with a discussion of death. But to sidestep the issue would be merely a pretense. Not everyone who has cancer will recover, no matter how brilliant the therapy.

In the words of spiritual healer Bruno Groening, quoted in the title pages of this report, "Any disease can be healed—but not every person".

Sometimes a person's time has come. None of us can escape the eventual sweep of the Grim Reaper's scythe. My concern, as a physician, is that people don't go to their graves before time, or with undue suffering. But no doctor, hospital or methodology can overthrow what God has set in place for that person.

Sometimes, try as we might, nothing seems to work and the patient declines inexorably. There is a strong sense that Fate has the upper hand. It does no good to bewail the circumstances and think it would all have been different "if only" (if only he or she had taken care of themselves better years ago; if only he or she had said they were experiencing symptoms; if only he or she had listened to advice.. and so on).

Sometimes the patient is his or her own worst enemy. It is very frustrating for family and friends to watch a person decline towards death, knowing there are workable strategies which could help (as given in this report). Yet the patient expresses no interest in trying extra tools for the job. Many is the time I have been called by distraught relatives and the conversation begins "My Mom (Dad, Aunt, Gran, Uncle, brother, whatever...) has terminal cancer. Can you help by advising me what they should do?"

Right at that moment I turn off the conversation and direct it back to the caller by saying "Is the patient interested in learning what alternatives are possible?" Nine times out of ten, there is a moment of hesitation and some kind of confession, like "I haven't actually told him/her I'm calling you".

The answer I'm sure you can guess: I always point out that it's a waste of time unless the patient is interested in helping in their own recovery. I always insist that the patient calls me.

Let's face it, most of the remedies and treatments I have been describing in this work are very demanding. I have even said that becoming a cancer patient is equivalent to a career shift. You have to do it 24 hours a day, indefinitely. It is always astonishing how many patients take the line that "I'd rather take my chances with the cancer than do all of that".

Well, we must respect the person's choice. Because it is all about choices. The aggressive and cruel system here in some states in the USA that makes it a requirement of law that a person can be forced against their wishes to undergo the blunderous brutality of conventional medicine should be anathema to all civilized societies.

Such laws, of course, are not based on compassion or any humanitarian motive but simply price fixing and are a violation of antitrust safeguards. Somehow the medical profession and drug industry has fooled the judiciary into believing they are above the law.

But enough of that. I'd like this to be a gentle, pastoral finish, as life itself should be.

I refer again to the words of famous oncologist and writer Bernie Siegel "Death is a kind of healing" (page 99). He's right. It is an end to suffering and often as much a relief for the survivors as to the demised. Yes, I am saying that relatives and friends too suffer horrendously when cancer visits.

The agonies suffered by those walking the final pathway with a terminally ill victim who lingers in pain are onerous to an unimaginable degree, until you have done it with someone you love.

It certainly helps to have some kind of supportive belief system, though I have seen even these collapse in the moments of extreme grief. When it happens to you, before your very eyes, it is easy to want to cry out "If there is a loving God, why did he allow this?"

Such reflections and the ultimate conclusions are, of course, beyond the scope of this report and outside my self-set remit. But I believe passionately that a doctor should care about these matters.

In the end, the best of physicians will introduce the salve of love and acceptance. No- one can go to their grave in peace if members of the family are torn to emotional shreds, believing that it is all some shocking outrage against Nature and reason.

Bear that in mind, always, and be gentle with your loved one as the lights finally go out. Your mission is to make it easy for them; THEN heal yourself.

Graceful Passages

As part of this close I would love here to introduce the work of my friend Gary Malkin. He is a brilliant composer (he has had several Emmy awards for his film music).

Gary has recorded an album of beautiful tracks with an end-of-life theme, accompanied by his gorgeous original music, called *Graceful Passages: A Companion for Living & Dying* (Gary Malkin and Michael Stillwater, 2000, New World Library). I know from many encounters with individuals that this combination of music and the spoken word has has been wonderfully healing and supportive for those facing the end. It works for both family and the patient.

Over 100,000 copies of this loving CD are in use throughout America and across the world, especially as an award-winning resource in hospice and clinic environments.

Graceful Passages is designed to help open the conversation around death and dying for anyone, but particularly for those facing it directly, helping to reduce anxiety about this last transition. It provides family members, patients, and health care providers with a spiritual sanctuary around the dying process.

One of the most beautiful and relevant tracks is by a man who faced cancer: 80-year old Lew Epstein. Lew is not an actor, he was not even rehearsed. Gary just asked him to speak from the heart. The results are quite magical: the gravelly voice of an elderly man who has learned what it means to face death and triumph—not in the immortality sense but in the overcoming of fear.

It is one of the most profound tracks on the whole album.

You can buy a set from Gary's website, with the Graceful Passages CD, an accompanying book of words and a second CD, called Unspeakable Grace, which is the same music but without the words. All that for $25. It is a great blessing, trust me.

Go here to get yourself a copy from Gary's "Wisdom Of The World" web-site:http://www.wisdomoftheworld.com/store/pc/viewPrd.asp?idpro-duct=4&idcategory=29